Reclaiming the Passion;

Stories that Celebrate
the Essence of Nursing

By Kristin Baird, RN, BSN, MHA

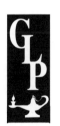 Golden Lamp Press

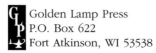 Golden Lamp Press
P.O. Box 622
Fort Atkinson, WI 53538

This is a non-fiction publication. Patient names have been changed to protect
confidentiality. Hospital or organization names may have been omitted for
confidentiality upon request of the interviewee or by discretion of the author.

Ordering Information
To order additional copies, contact your local bookstore, call (920) 563-4684
or log onto www.reclaimingthepassion.com. Quantity discounts are available.
ISBN 0-9754733-0-1 (paperback)

Library of Congress Cataloging-in-Publication Data

Baird, Kristin M., 1957-
    Reclaiming the Passion; Stories that Celebrate
  the Essence of Nursing   / Kristin M. Baird
      ISBN 0-9754733-0-1
      1. Nursing anecdotes   2. Motivation for nurses
      3. Love of nursing career   4. Baird, Kristin

Credits
      Developmental Editor: Rob Fixmer
      Proofreading and Copyediting: Bridget Baird
      Cover Design: Mark Dziewior

First printing: June 2004 (paperback)

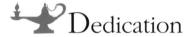

Dedication

This book is dedicated to the millions of nurses who make the world a better place through each and every encounter.

And to my parents, Robert and Audrey Fixmer, who always encouraged me to write and speak out about what I believe.

Contents

About the Author

Kristin Baird has over twenty-five years of experience in health care. Baird earned a BSN from the University of Wisconsin-Madison, and has clinical experience ranging from public health to critical care. She earned a Masters of Science in Health Services Administration from Cardinal Stritch College in Milwaukee.

Baird began consulting in 1991, specializing in health care marketing, communications and customer service. She has received more than twenty regional and national awards for health care writing, advertising, marketing and public relations.

Baird is the author of *Customer Service in Healthcare; A Grassroots Approach to Creating a Culture of Service Excellence* (2000. American Hospital Association Publishing and Jossey-Bass).

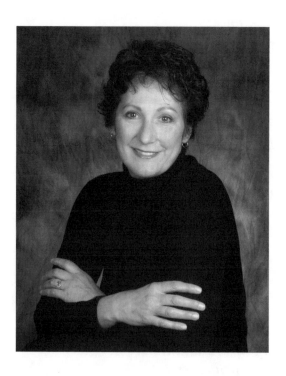

"The story — from Rumplestiltskin to War and Peace — is one of the basic tools invented by the human mind for the purpose of gaining understanding. There have been great societies that did not use the wheel, but there have been no societies that did not tell stories."

–Ursula K. LeGuin

⚱Preface

R eclaiming the Passion is the culmination of a process that spanned the better part of two decades. Working as a registered nurse gave me countless rich, personal experiences, not only with my patients and their families but with other nurses as well — nurses whom I admired and emulated and who probably never knew how much they influenced me. But the real seeds for the book were planted while I was still a nursing student at the University of Wisconsin-Madison. It was there that I was first exposed to the wonders of the nursing profession and to the pride we share in our work. It was also during those years that I began to see how little the outside world really knew about nursing. As with nearly everything in our culture, the media was shaping public opinion and attitudes about nursing. Movies and television so often portrayed us as half-wits and handmaidens that it's a wonder anyone of the post-TV generations ever entered the profession. While still a student, I vowed that someday I would help people understand the real work that nurses do.

Having worked in critical care, public health, community education, OB and as a call-center manager, I have countless nursing stories of my own. But at the time I was living the stories, I didn't truly appreciate that they were defining moments that helped both to shape a patient's experience and to mold my personal and professional development. I saw myself as a nurse on the job, just doing what I did. No big deal. Now, I believe that's part of our problem in nursing. It's why we're a misunderstood profession. Millions of us go to work every day in hospitals, clinics, nursing homes and home health settings throughout the world and see ourselves as "just a nurse," doing what any nurse would do. Well there is no such person as "just a nurse." You're the one making a difference, changing a life.

I came to this realization several years back while talking with my three daughters at the dinner table. When the subject turned to teen pregnancy — a subject all mothers of teens dread — I told them a story about a girl named Jenny.

She was only fifteen when she appeared on our OB unit in active labor, gum-snapping and sneering at her mother. Jenny sported a scull-and-crossbones tattoo and looked tough and hard beyond her years. After I escorted the pair to the birthing room, Jenny's mom turned to me and said, "She's all yours. I aint stickin' around for all the screamin'."

"As for you," she said pointing to Jenny, "now you'll see what you get for spreading your legs." With that, she turned and left.

Jenny sneered, rolled her eyes. "Figures," she said. "It's just like her to leave. I don't want her here anyway."

Jenny had received minimal prenatal care, and I knew from her admission interview that she planned to give the baby up for adoption. As tough as Jenny appeared when she arrived, I could tell she was frightened, and her bravado quickly faded with each contraction. Without prenatal classes, she was completely unprepared, and we had very little time to prepare her for the last stages of labor. With the help of the other nurses, I was able to spend nearly all my time with her. Toward the end, she was literally clinging to me and begging that I not leave her. Of course I couldn't. When my shift ended I called home to make last-minute child-care arrangements so I could stay with Jenny. She was terrified, and there was no way I was going to introduce a new nurse after we had established a level of trust.

When a mother makes the decision to give an infant up for adoption, we ask about her wishes for holding and looking at the baby. Each mother is different, but I always encouraged them to at least look at the baby in order to make the entire experience more real. If they hold the child, they can say goodbye in their own way.

Like many nurses, I never lose the sense of wonder at witnessing a birth. I am always in awe of the miracle and get teary-eyed every time. When the baby was delivered, the doctor announced it was a girl. Jenny openly wept and reached her arms out to me. "Will you please hold me?" she asked. "I just need someone to hold me." At that point, Jenny wasn't the only one crying. Everyone in the room was in tears. We held each other for a long time. And when she was ready, she allowed me to place her daughter in her arms for the combined mother-child introduction and farewell.

When I finished telling the story, my daughters were all in tears. "Oh my God, Mom! How can you do that?" one of them asked me.

I responded, "It's just what I do." But the minute the words left my lips, I realized that I was part of the problem. I was literally minimizing and discounting my work. Now, I want to be part of the solution. Helping nurses to tell their stories so that we, and the rest of the world will place greater value in this incredible profession.

In the process of creating this book, I have had the privelege of interviewing dozens of nurses who were willing to share their stories, and I found that the give and take of the interview process itself was crucial. Many of the best stories emerged only after encouraging nurses to dig far below the facts of a story to reveal their emotional responses, because inevitably it was the human aspects of a particular encounter or situation that helped to shape them as professionals. Together, we worked to divorce true emotion from mere sentimentality. The world has enough soap operas. I wanted the lessons learned in each story to emerge as an aggregate communal wisdom to be shared not only with other nurses but with readers from outside the profession who want to learn more about our work.

I learned very quickly that most people are intimidated by the thought of writing their own stories. If I had relied on nurses to commit their experiences to paper, I can guarantee that this book would never have been written. These remarkable stories would have remained locked inside these everyday heroes, and yet another generation would have no clue about the passion that energizes the nursing profession. Fortunately, nurses are generally willing, even eager, to talk about their experiences, even if they aren't sure they have a story to tell. Of course, they all do have stories. Oh, do they have stories!

But storytelling stems from the heart, while writing comes from the head. My role was to translate nurses' life experiences into written narratives by freeing them to open up and become storytellers. This is a key difference between *Reclaiming the Passion* and other collections of nurse's stories. The other crucial difference is that I am a registered nurse. I believe that having an informed view of nursing has been crucial in helping me establish the tone and theme of each story. They were written not to evoke sentimental reactions but rather to help other nurses reach back into their own memories for similar "aha!" moments.

Throughout this book, patients' names have been

changed to protect their privacy and to maintain professional confidentiality. Each nurse who agreed to be interviewed has reviewed and approved his or her story. Their credentials and current employers are listed where appropriate.

It is important to keep in mind that these are nurses you might find anywhere. True, some are in the high-tech, high-adrenaline nursing positions favored by television dramas and so-called reality shows. But most are the quiet heroes who nurture countless lives in clinics, hospitals, nursing homes and residential facilities all over the country each and every day. In these pages they share their shortcomings as well as their triumphs, but most importantly, they share the lessons they learned as real people following a path of professional development.

There are so many nurses out there. So many stories to be told. This is just a tiny snapshot of the big picture. But it's a start.

Kristin Baird
June 2004

"Never believe that a few caring people can't change the world. For, indeed, that's all who ever have."

–Margaret Mead

Acknowledgements

There have been so many people in my life who have supported my efforts at writing. But when I started this project I was overwhelmed by the generosity of time and talent that people were willing to share with me. I am still in awe of the encouragement I have received.

First and foremost, I want to thank my husband for not only the beautiful cover design but for his unwavering support. We met when he signed on as a designer for my consulting business. His designs and illustrations have always given life to my words, but his love gives depth to my life.

I would like to thank all of the nurses featured on the following pages. They indulged me with sometimes lengthy interviews. Some I knew personally, and some I had only the pleasure of "meeting" over the phone and Internet. Thank you for allowing me to document your experiences. I only hope that I have done you and your stories justice. The magnitude of your work is humbling.

Every writer needs a competent editor who can gently, but firmly guide a project. I am blessed to have a highly literary family which, when we pool our talents can cover the majority of writing and publishing challenges. I owe a world of gratitude to my editor and big brother, Rob Fixmer. With his help, I not only ended up with a clean manuscript but have learned so much about improving my style and technical skills.

My daughter Bridget Baird has been a Godsend to me over the past several months (actually the last twenty-four years but especially the last several months.) Her attention to detail has kept this project moving along so that I could focus my attention on writing and consulting.

My sister Elizabeth pitched in wherever she could to help find just the perfect quote to match every story. In spite of her own personal challenges in dealing with cancer, she always found time to read my stories and give me feedback.

My parents have encouraged all of their ten children to become better writers and communicators. Only in my maturity do I finally appreciate our lively dinner discussions about things like prepositional phrases and conjugating verbs. Who knew it would ever come in handy?

To Tammie Heintzman for sharing her gift of music with other nurses.

To Vivien De Back PhD, RN, for her timely feedback, which helped to make the book more interactive.

To Eleanor Sullivan, PhD, RN, whose review inspired confidence in the value of my work. Her mysteries as well as her academic publications enhance the image of nurses, and I am so honored by her praise.

To Kaye Lillesand RN, not only for her encouraging review, but for her leadership in nursing. Her pioneering work demonstrates that nursing really matters.

Above all, I want to thank the millions of nurses who are making the world a better place, one encounter at a time. Take the time to write, record and tell your stories. In doing so, you are helping to shape the profession. Love yourselves, and take time to celebrate your gifts.

"Live your life from your heart. And your story will touch and heal people's souls."

-Melody Beattie

Introduction

Maybe it was the time you stayed an extra five hours after your shift so an elderly patient wouldn't die alone. Perhaps it was the time you risked your job to stand up for a patient's rights. Or maybe it was the time a patient told you that just your presence made her feel better. Every nurse has moments when she is certain beyond a doubt that she has chosen the right profession. Those moments are like cool oasis waters, rich in their ability to rejuvenate and refresh the spirit. They are the points of passion that serve as an emotional counterbalance to the restrictive policies, stifling bureaucracies, staffing shortages and budget cuts that so often erode our souls. Our challenge is to rekindle the passion for caring and let it light the corners of our hospitals, clinics, nursing homes and, especially, our own lives. It is only when our spirits are rejuvenated that we can be our very best for our patients and ourselves.

Many of us can recall the first time we administered an injection, inserted an NG tube or started an IV. We can probably recount our first code blue or the first death or birth we witnessed. But how many critical events that have faded from our memories will be remembered forever by our patients? Many of us are so adept at balancing complex critical thinking with caring, compassion and little acts of kindness that such multitasking becomes second nature, so much a part of our work habits that we lose awareness of the emotional component. By minimizing our role (consciously or unconsciously) we fail to recognize the impact we have on others. While we cannot possibly recall every patient contact with any level of detail, chances are that our patients remember us, often vividly. Do they remember us for life-saving heroics? Perhaps, but much more likely they remember us for less dramatic, more human moments. Nursing is a juggling act that requires us to combine critical thinking and clinical skills with efficient organization, communication, compassion, negotiation and empathy. From the patient's perspective, it is often our nurturing interactions, rather than our cerebral feats, that are most memorable.

After all, health care settings are intimidating places. While a comfortable second home to nurses, they often terrify our patients. Sterile smells. Loud, intimidating machines. Alien terminology spoken by harried, uniformed professionals. Painful procedures and dehumanizing gowns. These are just a few of the "amenities" we offer. Patients are vulnerable, frightened and often in pain — both physically and emotionally — when they arrive at our clinics, hospitals or skilled nursing facilities.

Beyond that, we too often lose sight of the fact that some of a person's most life-altering moments happen in and around healthcare facilities. Traumatic injuries, major surgeries, grim diagnoses, death and birth are daily fare in a nurse's work environment.

Is it really any wonder that our patients clearly remember the nurse who stayed with them until a family member arrived after an accident? Or held their hand through a long, hard labor? Or brought a chocolate milk shake to celebrate a threshold crossed in physical therapy? Or presented their child with a cake when he was hospitalized on his birthday? These acts of kindness are all in a day's work for many nurses, but they are among the hallmarks of our profession.

I remember as a young nursing student feeling insulted when I heard people talk about nursing as a "calling or vocation." I resented any implication that nursing was a spiritual endeavor rather than a respected medical profession. I placed value on intellectual, scientific challenges, not on humanitarian aspirations. I laughed at a professor who encouraged students to become activists and advocates for nursing by quipping, "Ever since Florence Nightingale, we've been underpaid. It all started because she was carrying that damned lamp, which left only one hand free to collect the cash." While her comment may have been intended as harmless humor and while her motives were sincere, the unstated message was that our status as professionals was muddied by selfless acts of humanitarianism.

Today I see the missing logic in her viewpoint. Yes, we are educated. Yes, we are professionals worthy of a good salary and respect from our healthcare colleagues. But at the same time, the reason that most of us chose nursing over a laboratory setting was the desire to interact with people on a more personal and human level, where we could share in life on the front lines. The two are not mutually exclusive, nor should they ever be. We don't need to forego professional compensation just because we are compassionate. Nor should we apologize for embracing the very qualities that have made nursing a nurturing and holistic profession. For that we are extremely fortunate. We have the best of both worlds.

I never cease to be amazed at the countless qualities nurses bring to their work. Creativity, humor, compassion and generosity are just a few of the gifts shared between nurses and their patients. But sometimes I wonder, who is the true recipient of these gifts? Nurses learn so many of life's lessons from the experiences we share with our patients. Daily schooling in humility and judgment, in compassion and empathy, in human frailty and strength of spirit are just a few of the perks of our jobs.

Nursing is not a spectator sport. Day in and day out, we witness birth, death and all the traumas and challenges that life conjures in between. Along the way we become inured to the emotional dimensions of delivering care – so much so that many of us probably couldn't recall a single instance when our passion for nursing elevated the healing process beyond the mere delivery of medicine. And yet our days are rife with such examples. The problem is that we often must provide comfort and compassion as if on autopilot, and because a nurse typically cares for thousands of patients in the course of her career, the vast majority of their stories tend to meld in our memories or are lost altogether. Yet our actions and words are often etched forever in the memories of those whose lives we have touched.

As a consultant, I am often asked to do focus groups for my healthcare clients. One of my favorite ice breakers is to ask participants to identify their favorite healthcare character from TV or movies. It is rare that any of them mentions a nurse. More often than not they cite a doctor, even when the program they reference has prominent nurse characters. When nurses are mentioned, it is usually for some outrageous character trait rather than for leadership, competency or compassion. I cringe when Margaret "Hot Lips" Houlihan from *M*A*S*H* or Nurse Ratched from *One Flew Over the Cuckoo's Nest* are mentioned. While Margaret Houlihan is portrayed as a strong nurse leader, she is also painted as a flirtatious, neurotic sex object.

It's time that nurses tell their own stories. Rather than entrusting our image and purpose to screenplay writers, we can and should take the lead in defining ourselves and letting the world know what we do and what inspires us to do it. This collection of nurses' stories focuses not on life-saving heroics or clinical skills, but on tales of personal passion that reveal the real essence of nursing. But beyond inspirational reading, this book is intended to be an affirming, interactive process. For this reason, I have created a companion workbook/journal. (see the information on the back page of this book.) As you read through this collection of stories, use the workbook/journal to recall your own stories.

Many nurses struggle with articulating their stories, and sharing their experiences with small peer groups is a good way to become more comfortable with storytelling and through that process to enhance the service culture of your organization.

Through these stories I hope to leave other nurses with three things: to learn to tell their stories, to cherish their unique contributions and to reflect upon how their work helps to enrich lives — including their own.

"After silence, that which comes nearest to expressing the inexpressible is music."

–Aldous Huxley

Music for the Soul;

Tammie Heintzman shares her unique gifts with patients when they need her the most. As a hospice nurse in southern California, she works with families of patients who are struggling through their final days. From her first day as a hospice nurse in 1997, Tammie became overwhelmed with musical inspiration. As she met her patients and heard their stories, she discovered that their physical and emotional pain inspired inner melodies.

This was a new experience for Tammie, who had played piano for church and social events over the years but had never composed music. Grateful for the inspiration, she began recording the music and sharing it with her patients and families to promote relaxation and meditation.

Somewhere in the nursing school curriculum we become indoctrinated with rules about boundaries and professional conduct. "Don't get too close. Don't share personal information. Don't give or accept gifts." I am often concerned that many of these messages actually prevent nurses from reaching out on a more personal level, and thus experiencing the essence of what makes nursing a unique and human experience.

When asked if she grappled with some of the personal boundary issues, in sharing music with her patients, Tammie explained that at one point she had struggled with whether or not it was appropriate for her to be recording her piano music and giving tapes and CDs to her patients. In fact, at one point, her employer discouraged her from giving gifts of any sort.

"I think I considered his advice for about two seconds," she recalled. "Then I said, 'Well then, I can't work for

you. Sharing music is as much a part of their care as pain medication. If they don't want to listen, they don't have to, but if I can help ease their pain with music, I will.' And that was the end of the discussion."

Tammie's advice is simple. "Don't be afraid to share your gifts. Yes, it can feel risky to put yourself out there, because we all fear rejection and criticism. But the reality is that as nurses we have such a rare opportunity to share with people on a personal and human level."

In meetings and interviews, this gifted musician and healer shared countless stories about her patients and the music they have inspired in her. A CD of Tammie's original piano compositions is enclosed with the companion journal, Journaling to Reclaim the Passion.

Morning Song

"The Morning Song" was inspired by a 50-year-old man with cancer. Suffering with intense pain and a dismal diagnosis, Jim addressed everyone around him harshly, including me, his new hospice nurse. I remember him snarling, "Just do what you have to do here, and get it over with." It was evident he was using all of his inner resources just coping with physical and emotional pain.

At the end of my first visit with the family, Jim's wife, Peggy, followed me out to my car to apologize profusely for Jim's behavior. I told Peggy there was no need to apologize. While we sat talking in my car, Peggy asked what CD was playing. Not revealing that it was one of my own untitled compositions, I handed Peggy the CD and suggested that she play it to help Jim relax and cope with his pain.

The next day Jim greeted me with open arms. He was

so grateful to have the music and talked about how it had helped him through a rough night. We talked throughout my visit, and I felt that we were truly connecting. Unlike the day before, Jim was talkative and enthusiastic. I mentioned that I had seen a beautiful orange and black bird outside my window that morning. He told me that what I had seen was an oriole and talked on about his interest in birds. As we talked, an oriole lit on the feeder outside his window as if to confirm my earlier sighting.

Almost immediately I began hearing piano music in my head. I know that sounds very strange, and I always hesitate to tell people about how my musical compositions come to me. But I have learned over the years that when I am inspired with a song, I just have to give in, sit down at the piano and play it. This time was no different.

Immediately upon returning home, I sat down at the piano and composed a song that I dedicated to Jim. I recorded the piece and brought the CD to him the next day.

Jim took his CD to the hospital with him a few days later when he was admitted and diagnosed with metastasis to the pancreas. Peggy later told me, "He listened to that CD over and over and over. You just wouldn't believe how many doctors and nurses were moved to tears by your music. We've also noticed that Jim's vital signs show a real calmness when his song is playing."

Jim never left the hospital, and we all felt a sense of relief knowing that his struggle with cancer had ended. Just knowing that my music could help him to cope with his pain was incredibly rewarding. Jim's family thanked me effusively for sharing my music with them, but what they could never understand was that I was the true recipient of a gift. They had honored me by allowing me to share with them. I was actually just giving them back their song.

Gentle Flight

It was Easter weekend in 2000 when I was first asked to visit Donald. After battling cancer for six months, Donald had just been told he had only about three weeks to live. A highly successful business man, he lived with his wife, Mary, in a very affluent area of town. Mary, who had never worked outside of the home, had become Donald's caregiver when he could no longer care for himself. Donald, always the hard-driving businessman, tended to bark orders at home in the same way he had as CEO of his corporations.

When I arrived at their home for the first time, Donald was talking to a financial adviser on the phone and had an attorney and an accountant in the living room. During more than fifty years of marriage, Mary had never been involved in his business and had never handled more money than her grocery and household funds. When Donald learned he was dying, he arranged to have these professionals on board to help his wife understand his business and holdings.

When I first encountered Donald, he was telling Mary, "So there, I don't want any argument. I love you and I've made arrangements to go to a nursing home to die. Life goes on in this home. I'm not going to die here."

To anyone else, his words would have seemed gruff, but I saw them as his final gift to his wife. By making arrangements for his own care and for Mary's financial well-being, Donald was trying to care for her even after he was gone. He showed no softness on the surface, but I sensed that deep down he was a caring man who truly loved his wife.

Almost immediately upon witnessing this interaction, I

began hearing this song starting in my head. When I am inspired like this, it is as though I have put headphones on. The music gets louder and louder if I don't just give into it. After leaving Donald and Mary's house, I returned home to compose and record the song that had been running through my mind.

When Donald was admitted to a skilled nursing facility the next day, he and Mary both knew he would never return home. Although I was no longer involved in his care, I visited him at the nursing home and brought the CD I had recorded for him. Not having a well established relationship with Donald, I felt a little uneasy about my visit but thought I would take a chance. Handing him the CD, I explained that he had inspired me with his bravery and his desire to care for his wife's needs.

Here was a man who was accustomed to a level of luxury most of us will never know. Yet he listened to the music in total awe, then turned to me and asked, "We inspired this?" With tears in his eyes he took my hands and thanked me. "This is such a wonderful gift," he said. "I can't believe you would do this for me."

I had no choice but to give this music to Donald. It was his. This man had just about everything that money could buy, but he couldn't buy more time. I had been so moved by this hard-driving man whose life had been centered on logic. He had made such a gentle plan for comforting his wife. Saying goodbye to him, I wished him a gentle flight.

Velvet Curtain

M aggie was in her fifth bout with breast cancer, and the doctors weren't giving her much hope when I started hospice visits. A young mom, barely forty, Maggie had always been full of life and optimism. After so many remissions during the past six years, Maggie's life had been something of a roller coaster. The one constant throughout her entire cancer ordeal was her 7-year-old daughter Molly. I really think it was Molly who gave Maggie the will to keep on fighting.

When Maggie started to hit a downhill slide and required more care, we spent more and more time together. She was always so undemanding about her care and rarely asked for anything, but one day she said, "Tammie, I need your help with something."

Surprised that she would finally ask anything of me, I quickly responded, "Anything. Anything at all. What is it?"

Her request was anything but a small one. "I just don't know how to tell Molly that I won't be in her life as she grows up. I don't know how to say that she'll go to middle school, high school and college without me there to support her. I don't know how to say the words or to help her cope," she said with tears in her eyes. "I just don't know what to say or how to say it."

Not knowing how to respond immediately, I told Maggie that I needed to think about this. I had absolutely no idea what I would do if faced with a similar challenge. I, too, was a young mother with two daughters and couldn't begin to imagine how I would discuss this issue with them.

Pondering our discussion later that evening, I sat down at my piano. Music has always been soothing and meditative stress relief for me, especially since I became a hospice nurse. On that particular evening, while thinking about little Molly and her mom's difficult task ahead, a song came to me. As I played the song I decided that it was meant for Molly, so I recorded it onto a cassette tape.

Not having any profound words of wisdom for Maggie yet, I explained that in my own family, music was a very calming and meditative influence, not just for adults but for my daughters as well. I explained that music had been one of the most important coping tools my daughter used in dealing with the sudden, accidental death of our neighbor and that, if it was okay, I would like to give Molly some music that might encourage her to get quiet and listen to her feelings. Maggie agreed, and I gave the tape to Molly during my next visit. I explained that the tape was special music just for her. I told her that if she wanted to, she could take the tape to her room, get real quiet and just listen to it. She eagerly took the tape, and as I was leaving I heard her playing the recording.

The next day Molly told me how the music had affected her. She summed up her emotions as only a 7-year-old could. "Tammie, my music was so pretty, but so sad. Whenever I listen to it, I just pull my covers up over my head and cry and cry and cry."

I hadn't intended to evoke raw grief, and I think my expression must have shown. Before I could even open my mouth to apologize for creating an emotional upheaval, Maggie reached out and took my hand and said, "Thank you, Tammie, this is exactly what we needed. In her own way, Molly knows that we are reaching the end. And what we both really needed was to just curl up in bed, pull the covers over our heads and cry and cry and cry together. Your music helped us to find a way to do just that. Molly invited me into her bed to just cry with her. It opened the door for us to start talking about everything we needed to talk about. Thank you."

Without realizing it on a conscious level, I had been mentally naming this composition, The Velvet Curtain. How appropriate that it be named this. With the help of their very own Velvet Curtain, Maggie and Molly were able to shut out the rest of the world surrounded by the rich, luxurious softness of each others' arms.

The real lesson I have learned from all of this is that we cannot be afraid to share with our patients. As nurses we are taught to keep a professional distance, but I disagree. We have to embrace the human side of our experiences. Yes, it can be emotionally risky, but I say go for it. Life is so much more rewarding when you do.

As told by:
Tammie Heintzman, RN
Palliative Care Nurse
San Diego, California

Piano compositions entitled Velvet Curtain, Gentle Flight and Morning Song can be found on the companion CD included with Journaling to Reclaim the Passion, or on Tammie's website www.touchrecords.com

To think about and journal

Think about times when you have shared your unique gifts with your patients. Record your thoughts and memories in Journaling to Reclaim the Passion in the section entitled "Sharing your Gifts".

"Constant attention by a good nurse may be just as important as a major operation by a surgeon"

–Dag Hammarshkjold

🕯A Change in Priorities

Nearly every nurse I have ever met has a story about a single patient who changed the course of her career and put her life's work into perspective. Maureen Gosser's story is an example of how priorities change when we listen carefully.

I t was my first job after graduation, and I prided myself in efficiency and technical skills. At the large teaching hospital in the Midwest where I was working, I was wowed by the technology and impressed by the staff's credentials and the hospital's reputation. Like many of the nurses on my unit, I was convinced that our efficiency and technical skills were the assets of greatest value to our patients. Then I met Gert.

It was Thanksgiving Day, and I had approached my shift with my usual zeal and organization — a list of patients and a list of well-organized tasks to be completed in a timely fashion.

Gert was in her nineties and had recently undergone a total hip replacement. I had cared for her the day before, and I realized I had not seen any visitors with her. When I finished her vital signs, IV and incision site check, Gert patted the side of her bed and asked me to sit with her. "I just want to talk a little while, dear," she said.

Clearly Gert had no idea how busy I was. My list of important tasks was nearly burning a hole in my pocket. Gently, but firmly, I told her I was too busy to just sit and talk. But Gert persisted, to the point of nearly begging me to sit with her. After my third refusal, Gert pulled out her purse and said, "I will pay you five dollars if you will just sit and talk with me for a while."

I was devastated. In my rush to get my scheduled tasks checked off, I had failed to see what this patient really needed from me. All she wanted was a little time and attention, and I had discounted her. She was lonely and spending the holiday in a hospital, and all I could focus on was my 'to do' list. I left the room but immediately re-arranged my list of priorities to allow me the time to come back and sit with Gert for a little while.

To this day, I cry when I think back on that experience. Gert taught me an important lesson about balancing priorities with patients' needs. Nursing care isn't always about medical care. Sometimes the most important thing we can give our patients is just a few minutes to let them know we value them as human beings. Five dollars was a fortune to a woman in her nineties, but she was willing to give it to me in exchange for a little time and compassion. Now I make sure I find a few extra moments with my patients just to listen and be present with them. It's amazing how many tasks on the 'to do' list can be re-arranged when we make listening a priority.

As told by:
Maureen Gosser, RN

To think about and journal

Think about lessons you have learned throughout your life about the value of being productive vs. the value of taking time for relationships. Does one have greater value than the other? What lessons were emphasized in your nursing education?

Turn to "Setting Priorities" in *Journaling to Reclaim the Passion for additional reflection.

* *Turn to Page 178 for a brief description of Journaling to Reclaim the Passion.*

"Nobody cares how much you know, until they know how much you care."

–Theodore Roosevelt

✺ Efficiency isn't Enough

Sharon Chinn entered nursing school after first completing a degree in bacteriology from UCLA. Recognized as one of the most organized and efficient nurses on her pediatric rehab unit, Sharon was often praised by peers and managers alike for her abilities. But she had a rude awakening one day when she realized there was much more to being a good nurse than meeting a schedule.

Early in my career I felt that being a good nurse meant getting tasks done correctly and on time. I would start my shift by getting report, then prioritize my day by organizing tasks. I always felt a sense of gratification as I made my rounds and checked off the tasks from my list. I was regarded by my manager and peers as an extremely efficient team member. However, I was about to discover that priding myself on efficiency had made me appear cold and uncaring.

It was about one year after I began working on a pediatric rehab unit that I had my career-altering encounter. I had been caring for Tommy, a 20-month-old with a diagnosis of herpes encephalitis. Tommy's infection was neurologically devastating. He couldn't eat, sit or even roll over. Once a bright child with limitless potential, Tommy was now agitated, disoriented and unable to recognize his own mother. He could no longer eat normally and required an NG tube for his every-four-hour feedings.

During my regular shifts, I would go into Tommy's room, greet his mother, take his vital signs, check the NG and inspect the skin around the tube. During this process I would always explain to his mother what I was doing.

Looking back on these encounters, I considered myself friendly but efficient and professional in the care of all my patients, and Tommy was no exception.

This said, I was stunned when his mother stopped me in the hallway outside of his room. "I don't want you taking care of Tommy anymore," she said. "You come in, do what you have to do, and move on to the next patient. I realize that you have a lot of patients, but my baby is so sick. He needs more care than you are giving him. I want his nurses to care about him, hold him and touch him. You just don't do that for him."

I was devastated. No one had ever so much as implied that I was giving substandard care. My meds were always administered on time and with the greatest accuracy. My assessment skills were excellent, and I took pride in making sure I was always on top of the latest literature in pediatric rehab. My manager and peers could always count on me to get the job done, so who was this woman to insult me like this?

My first instinct was to argue with her. I wanted to say, "OK, I can sit and rock Tommy, but how happy would you feel if his meds were late or if his four-hour feedings weren't done on schedule?" But I didn't say any of those things. Hurt and insulted, I remember asking myself if I was cut out to be a pediatric nurse after all. Maybe I didn't have what it takes.

But rather than wallow in my anger and hurt, I took this mother's words to heart and spent time reflecting on what had just happened. My most important realization was that I had not acknowledged how devastating the diagnosis had been for this family. The hopes and dreams they had held for Tommy only a few short weeks before had been shattered by a destructive viral infection. There was no way this mother could know what kind of future was in store for her son. While her expectation for a positive outcome eroded, the most she could hope for was kindness and attention from all of us who were caring for Tommy.

It became clear to me that while I had been interacting with Tommy and his mom in a friendly yet efficient manner, I had not been taking the extra couple of seconds to really look at the mom and to ask how she was doing. In caring for Tommy, I had not shown that I cared about him as a person or about a member of his family in crisis. I hadn't been touching, talking to, or interacting with the boy. Of course I cared about him, but I realized I hadn't been demonstrating it in a way that felt supportive and loving to the family. I knew I didn't want my other patients or their families to see me the way this mother did.

The next day I returned to the unit and stopped in to see Tommy and his mother. I thanked her for being candid with me about how she viewed my nursing care. I acknowledged that I had been missing a critical part of Tommy's care and had not been sensitive enough to her needs. I apologized and reiterated my thanks for her candor. She clearly was touched by our conversation, and she allowed me to continue caring for her son.

Looking back, I can honestly say I was blessed that someone pointed this out to me early in my career. I had received so many pats on the back for my efficiency and technical skills that I had started to emphasize those qualities more than the compassionate elements of nursing. The children on our unit were coping with physically and emotionally devastating conditions. In addition to providing astute physical care, I needed to be more in tune with the emotional and psychological needs of the families who were trying to cope with this devastation.

It wasn't until several years later, when I had a sick

child of my own, that I could truly understand what I had missed. My daughter, Stephanie, was born at 31 weeks gestation and needed to spend weeks in the neonatal intensive care unit (NICU). I was distraught with fears about what the future might hold for her. Stephanie was my third child, and I had always considered the postpartum period to be an exciting time, but now I was facing sheer terror as she struggled through her first days.

I immediately recognized how sensitive the nurses were being to my emotional needs. Without saying anything, they had admitted me to a bed on the postpartum unit that was far away from the other new moms. Later I realized that they wanted to give me that physical space so that I didn't have to mingle with mothers who were excitedly chatting about their healthy newborns; inevitably, they would have been asking me about my baby.

The nurses recognized that I needed space and time to adjust to my unforeseen turn of events. They didn't say anything about their decision to separate me from the others; they just did it without making a big deal about it. I didn't hear the other babies or have to be awakened as a roommate breastfed in the middle of the night. Literally everyone on the staff who interacted with me; the aide, housekeeper, nurses, and dietary staff alike, knew that my baby was in NICU. Each person would enter and ask how my baby was doing. They were all very supportive.

I was afraid and had no idea what the future would hold for my daughter. I asked a lot of questions – so many that at one point, I actually apologized to the medical director of the NICU for being so inquisitive. His response will stay with me forever. "Please don't apologize for asking so many questions," he said. "I know that your daughter is the most important person in the world to you." His compassion and understanding were exactly what I needed at the time, and it served as a lesson I was able to apply to my nursing practice. Suddenly I understood firsthand the value of a personal connection with patients and their families.

When I later became the manager of the unit where I had once cared for Tommy and his mother, I shared my perspective-changing lesson with every new staff member during her orientation. I stressed that what they did while on the unit was their job, but for these families, the rest of their life would be tied up in the care of their children. It's not just a clean bed, vitals and meds on time that make a good nurse.

Although I know I can never get inside the body and mind of someone else, this experience helped me to recognize what is most important to a family dealing with crisis. It's that personal connection that matters. When we take that little bit of extra time to connect with a patient, to show respect for him or her as a human being and compassion for a family in crisis, we are moving from ordinary to extraordinary care.

As told by:
Sharon Chinn, RN

To think about and journal

Was there a time when you may have placed tasks above human relationships? Refer to "Setting Priorities" in Journaling to Reclaim the Passion *for memory joggers on this subject.*

"If you can learn from hard knocks you can also learn from soft touches."

-Carolyn Kenmore.

The Art of Nursing

Since beginning her nursing career in the early 1960s, Karen Lee Fontaine has witnessed profound changes in the profession. Troubled by the shift away from the art of healing toward a much greater emphasis on technology and science, Karen has written several books and articles that help nurses discover value in traditional healing practices, beginning with simple human touch. There is no doubt that solid technical knowledge is the basis of safe nursing practice, but it is the art of nursing that is truly the soul of the profession.

I n the early 1960s when I started my career, patient acuity was significantly less than it is today, which allowed for much longer hospital stays. This gave the nursing staff an opportunity to spend more time getting to know our patients. One of the fondest memories I have from my early nursing career was working the PM shift. A team of us would make bedtime rounds, giving each patient a backrub and tucking them in for the night. Those comfort measures still stand out in my mind as one of the most gratifying elements of nursing care.

But the entire profession has experienced a pronounced shift. Today there is a much greater emphasis on science and technology in the nursing curriculum and a shift away from the true art of nursing. As a professor, I can understand how the shift occurred, because there is so much to learn in such a short period of time. But the art of nursing is being forsaken for the science of medicine. The art that I speak of has to do with our ability to be truly present for our patients and to employ nurturing and healing acts, beginning with simple touch. Ultimately, art versus science comes down to the difference between healing versus curing our patients. Healing is based on art whereas curing is anchored in science. We're not being fair to ourselves when we minimize the value of the art that is the soul of our profession.

Part of the shift that we are witnessing is due to the educational process. It seems that so many students enter the program because they are caring and compassionate and truly desire to help others, but we end up "teaching" those qualities right out of them. The learning curve in nursing education is very steep, given the increasingly sophisticated technology and complex health problems. It seems there is little time or energy left over for anything else. Even the board exams are upping the ante. It used to be that students graduated and worked in med/surg for a year to establish a strong foundation before moving into specialty areas. But today, with the nursing shortage, students are graduating and moving right into critical care, emergency nursing and other once restricted areas. The board exams, therefore, have had to change to assess competencies in all these areas.

I am seeing another change in nursing students that I have not seen in the past. Now, more than ever, people are entering nursing in search of a steady job and financial security. I know this is a gross generalization, but I see a little less of the commitment and passion that I saw years ago. Of course, I still get many committed students entering the program, but I am seeing a significant rise in the security seekers who don't have a true passion for the profession. Again, at the risk of generalizing, I find that the nontraditional students seem to be more caring. But I also realize that we do something to our students in nursing school. There is so much content that learning becomes pressured. Students go from pressured learning to pressured jobs. We don't take time to teach students to just be present for their patients. We don't place enough value on helping them to be comfortable spending time and reaching out to patients. I tell my students, "If you walk into a room and focus on the machine, you are nursing the machine and not the human attached to it." And that is really what happens. Technology has caused us to focus first on the machine that's beeping and not the human attached to that machine.

Still, I am optimistic, because many of us in the academic world are coming to this realization and are trying to refocus on the art of healing in our teaching. That shift has required an immense change in philosophy and one that has not been embraced with open arms by the more traditional nursing curriculum directors. I know I don't have all the answers, but I try to lead by example and with my own enthusiasm.

Because I feel so strongly about getting back to the art of nursing, I have developed a course in alternative medicine. Nursing as a caring profession embraces philosophical perspectives similar to those of many alternative healing systems and therapies. My desire is to help students see nursing from a broader perspective. Nurses using the healing model, in contrast to the curing model, allow themselves to be everything they already are and move toward a greater sense of the meaning of their experiences.

One thing I try to stress is the patient's right to choose his or her own path. I hate the term non-compliant, because it means the patient isn't obeying us, when in reality they may be simply choosing a different path from the one that traditional medicine prescribes for them. I teach an introduction to nursing course, and it is so much fun because I get to witness the raw, unbridled enthusiasm of the students before they have been "molded" by science and technology. They're fresh, ready to take it all in and, frankly, not yet burned out.

A revelation that caused my own paradigm shift occurred a few years ago when my partner was battling leukemia. I walked into his hospital room where he lay drained and listless — emotionally and physically. He asked that I lie with him, hold him and send him some of my healing energy. My heart knew this was what he needed, but my head was sending out the conflicting messages I had learned in nursing school. "Never sit on a patient's bed. This is their private space and you must never cross that boundary." Crawling into bed with him was against everything I had learned as a nurse. But I did it anyway and continued doing it every day while he was in the hospital. Each time I lay with him he told me that he could feel his strength building from our shared energy. He told me that sharing my energy was the most comforting thing that anyone could do for him.

In the room next door to my partner was an elderly couple in their seventies. The wife was dying. As I passed by her room day after day, I could see the helplessness on her husband's face as he held her hand, keeping the polite distance. Now, here was a couple who had probably been sleeping in the same bed for more than fifty years, and nothing about our hospital atmosphere supported this man doing what was surely in his heart. I wanted so badly to tell him to just crawl into that bed and hold her for the last time. But I didn't, because I wasn't a nurse in that hospital and felt I would be overstepping my bounds. I fear that their distance left them both with some unfinished business.

A few months later, when my mother was dying, there was little I could do to relieve her pain, but I knew I could comfort her. I lay on her bed and just held her as she died. It brought us both peace and closure.

So much research has been done on the value of therapeutic touch and yet we put up these barriers. The concept of Therapeutic Touch derived from nursing so why aren't we teaching this? The essence of what we have to offer our patients is nurturing and comforting, but the art of healing is sacrificed for the dominant curriculum in technology and science. I'm not saying that students don't need to learn about science and technology, because they do. But art and science don't have to be mutually exclusive.

Along with others, I have made a personal commitment to bringing a greater balance between the art and science of our curriculum at Purdue University. I have developed a course for nurses on alternative medicine. It has become very popular and fills up faster each semester. I find that students are intrigued and hungry for more information about alternative therapies for healing. We spend time meditating during every class period and I ask them to keep a journal to document their thoughts and feelings as we explore a variety of healing arts.

Although it isn't a hands-on clinical, the students are exposed to massage and a multitude of complementary and alternative therapies. According to their journals I find that many of them are already beginning to apply the philosophies in their clinical settings. It wasn't easy introducing alternative medicine into the curriculum. I had to fight the faculty to get the course approved originally, and now it is counted as a nursing science elective. We have a long way to go to rediscover the value in the art of nursing, but it's a beginning. And I'm glad to be a part of it.

As told by:
Karen Lee Fontaine, RN, MSN, Professor of Nursing
Purdue University Calumet

Karen Lee Fontaine is the author of eleven texts including *Mental Health Nursing 5th ed (2003 Prentice Hall)* and Healing Practices, *Alternative Therapies for Nurses (2000, Prentice Hall)*. A second edition will be released under the title *Complimentary and Alternative Medicine for Nurses* in 2005.

🪔Finding Peace

Nursing education seems to place so much emphasis on the skills we need to preserve life that we enter the profession ill-prepared to deal with death. It is only with experience and maturity that we become comfortable with the myriad emotions surrounding death. As Laurie Purtell discovered, death can mean relief not only from physical pain but from emotional suffering as well.

I had been working as an ICU nurse in our community hospital for about two years when I was called from the unit to help out in the ER. There had been a fatal automobile accident not far from the hospital; two were dead at the scene and two more were in critical condition.

The accident had occurred early on a Monday morning when a man I'll call Jack was dropping off his two children, one at school, the other at daycare. When his car hit the gravel along the shoulder of the highway, Jack became startled. He overcorrected, swerved and headed right into oncoming traffic. Among the two people dead at the scene was his 5-year-old son. His 8-year-old daughter was in critical condition and had to be airlifted to a trauma center.

Although Jack had suffered trauma that included a shattered pelvis, he never lost consciousness. He continually asked about his children. The ER physicians explained that his daughter had been air-lifted to a trauma center and that his wife had been called. In spite of his constant questions, the doctor felt it best to withhold the news that his son had been killed.

When I arrived in the ER, Jack was my main focus. The doctor had told me during my brief report that it was best not to tell Jack of his son's death yet, but now Jack was pleading with me for information about the boy. I took the doctor aside and told him, "You have got to tell this man about his son. He deserves to know." Reluctantly, the physician went to Jack's bedside where he told him the heartbreaking news.

As I held Jack's hands, he looked me in the eyes and said, "You have to shoot me. I just can't live. This is all my fault."

I don't remember my exact words, but I know I said something like, "You need to be strong. This is so hard, but you have to hold on for your wife and daughter." At times like these there are really no words of comfort, no matter how hard we try.

Looking into Jack's face, I swear that I saw something leave in his eyes. It was as if his very spirit was being pulled out of him. If the will to live is manifested as the sparkle in someone's eyes, I saw it vanish from him at that precise moment. I knew in my heart that he could not live with the anguish of losing his son and feeling responsible.

Within minutes of our discussion, Jack's wife arrived in the ER. I was sick at her reaction on a number of levels. The pain she must have felt didn't surface as grief, but only as anger and blame. Standing over Jack's bed, she just kept saying, "What have you done? What have you done?" I could see that he was emotionally destroyed.

The complexities of Jack's injuries required that he, too, be airlifted to a trauma center within the hour. I never saw Jack again, but two days later I read his obituary in the paper. He had died of an embolism.

He was young, so I suppose I should have felt sad, but instead I felt relieved. I just thought, This is truly the grace of God. I really don't think he could have lived with the guilt and pain of his loss. I took comfort in knowing he was with his son.

As nurses, we seem to go through phases of learning to cope with death. Over time, we come to anticipate and welcome death when patients are suffering with physical pain. This was the first time I had felt a sense of comfort knowing that in death a patient had escaped what would surely have been a lifetime of regret and emotional pain.

As told by:
Laurie Purtell, RN

"Act quickly, think slowly,"

- Germaine Greer

Don't Blow it

Being in a hurry doesn't mean we can afford to leave our brains on hold. Doug Egdorf shared a funny vignette that proves that regardless of our workload, we need to keep our brains attached to our actions at all times.

I was orienting a new nurse on our med/surg unit and it was one of those days when you feel like you're meeting yourself coming and going down the hall. I had left the nurse-in-training to apply a condom catheter on one of our patients and just as she applied the adhesive, his IV ran out. As I walked into the room, my eyes nearly popped out of my head at the spectacle before me. In her rush to get to the IV, she started blowing on the adhesive to hasten the drying process. Need I say more?

As told by:
Doug Egdorf, RN, BSN
Emergency Nurse

"Let us touch the dying, the poor, the lonely and the unwanted according to the graces we have received, and let us not be ashamed or slow to do the humble work."

–Mother Teresa

⚘Honoring What is Sacred

There are so many situations in nursing that require us to look past policies and procedures in order to do what is right for the patient and family. Suzanne Marnocha's story demonstrates how rich our own experiences can be when we step back and let families and patients take the lead.

One morning when I reported for work in the ICU, my care partner reported that one of our patients had already died. My colleague had been through a terribly rough night, so I said she should just turn the patient over to me for post-mortem care. I didn't know the patient at all, but I knew that her daughter and several women from their church were present.

Cynthia was only in her fifties and had died after a massive heart attack. As I approached her bedside, the group sitting with her was quiet but they openly welcomed me. In fact, they seemed grateful that I was there. I explained what I needed to do for Cynthia's post-mortem care. I described the process for removing the tubes and lines and for bathing her. When the women said they would like to help me with this process, I was taken aback. Rather than accepting their offer, I said I needed to call my supervisor. It sounds so silly now that I felt a need to check with my supervisor, but it felt awkward at the time.

When I think back on that day, I now realize that these women were Cynthia's daughter and closest friends. Why wouldn't they have the right to do what they felt they needed to do to prepare her body for the funeral director? In reality, they should have had more rights than me or any other health care professional at that point.

When I returned to Cynthia's bedside, the group was singing and praying around her. There was no wailing or overt grief, just a peaceful, almost joyful acceptance. As I grew a bit more comfortable with the women, I brought basins of water for them to bathe Cynthia. I was a little nervous about taking out the sutures and removing the intra-aortic balloon with them present because those procedures can be pretty ugly. But the women stayed for the entire process and talked with me about her spirit leaving her body. It was a beautiful experience.

The loving and respectful way they handled Cynthia made me think about how the women prepared Jesus' body for the tomb and I was reminded how other stories from the Bible also describe rituals that included the cleansing of the body in preparation for burial.

That morning, we had started out as strangers, and yet I felt they had included me in something very personal and spiritual.

The experience taught me that we, as nurses, need to encourage families to be more involved in the care of their loved ones. I think families often hold back and wait for "permission" from us to minister to the needs of their loved ones. We can learn and experience so much when we step back at times and let the family take the lead. My initial hesitation derived from concerns about hospital policy rather than from a concern about the needs of the family. If I had forbidden these caring women from getting involved, we would have all missed out on a rich and meaningful experience.

As told by:
Suzanne Marnocha, RN MSN PhD CCRN.
Assistant Professor
University of Wisconsin-Oshkosh

To think about and journal

Reflect on an experience where you have needed to step back and allow patients and family members to exercise rituals or traditions unfamiliar to you. What did you learn about cultural or religious traditions different from your own?

Turn to "Spiritually Speaking" in <u>Journaling to Reclaim the Passion</u> for further reflection.

"Teach this triple truth to all: A generous heart, kind speech and a life of service and compassion are the things that renew humanity."

–Buddha

"The Feeling"

Good nursing is a balance between the science of medicine and the art of caring for another human being. Critical thinking skills can be developed over one's career, but intuition is innate. Most nurses I know agree that intuition or gut instincts about our patients are almost never wrong. When Maureen Gosser first experienced "the feeling" as a young nurse, and reluctantly acted on it, she learned two crucial lessons — about herself and about the line between compassion and professional responsibility.

When 80-year-old Vince arrived on our surgical unit as a fresh post-op, I was ready for him. I knew he'd had a history of diabetes, and had just undergone an amputation below the knee. Checking in briefly with the recovery room nurse, I felt confident in his condition and left the room to chart. If all went well, I would be able to take my dinner break as scheduled.

I was a new grad in a large, reputable teaching hospital and wanted to impress my senior team members. Thus far, I had done a pretty good job. I was quickly gaining a reputation as a bright and efficient nurse worthy of their trust and respect. But that day, and on that shift, when I sat down to chart, I was suddenly overcome with "the feeling" that something wasn't right. Now, after having been a nurse for two decades, I have come to know and respect "the feeling," but that was the first time I had ever experienced it. I just knew in my gut that something wasn't right with Vince. Since there was no way I could ignore the nagging sensation, despite every clinical indication, I returned to his room. Lo and behold, I found Vince pale, diaphoretic and gasping for air.

I whipped back the covers and discovered that he was hemorrhaging. There was blood everywhere beneath that cover sheet. He was already barely responsive. With one hand, I grabbed the hemorrhage site, and with the other, I pushed the call button. Within seconds, a team was at my side preparing to return Vince to surgery. In the face of all the clinical heroics surrounding his bed, Vince grabbed me, looked directly into my eyes and said, "Please let me die. I just want to die. Now."

Vince was pleading with me through clear eyes and a completely articulate tongue, "I just want to die," he told me with conviction. At that moment, he was whisked from the room and off to surgery by the crash team. I thought "Oh my God! Who are we to go against this man's wishes? He wants to die, and I just sent him off to surgery."

He returned to our unit once the hemorrhage was stopped, but I never again saw the kind of animation I had witnessed when he was begging to die. In fact, when I talked to him, he turned away and avoided eye contact with me at any cost.

I was terribly distressed by that incident. I had encountered several life-and-death moments by that time in my career, yet I had never been asked to just let someone die. Who was I to make a judgment call that would determine this man's fate to decide how his life should end? Should he not be able to decide when enough was enough?

I was barely twenty years old. How could I possibly know what was in this man's best interest? Struggling with all of these questions, I was truely questioning whether or not I was suited for nursing. But when I met with my supervisor to seek her counsel, she had the wisdom and sensitivity to help me sort through my uncertainties.

"You absolutely did the right thing," she told me. "It is not acceptable to let a patient bleed to death on a surgical floor."

I thought about it and had to agree. Yes, it was Vince's right to want to die, but he had consented to surgery and had placed himself into our care. At that point, I was not responsible for of his decision. I had no choice but to follow our course of treatment.

Logic aside, this was a terribly difficult time for me, especially since Vince would never again look at me. But I walked away from the experience with two important lessons. First was that every patient has the right to die, but we need to follow accepted medical procedures. Second, and probably most important, I should never ignore "the feeling," the little voice that tells me something is wrong. In twenty-two years of nursing, that voice has never been wrong.

As told by:
Maureen Gosser, RN

To think about and journal

Have you ever been faced with a conflict between a patient's desires and acceptable protocol? Record your thoughts, memories and feelings about those situations in the journal under, "Between a Rock and a Hard Place".

Think about times when a gut feeling has prompted you in decisions about a patient. Turn to "Gut Feelings" in the Journaling to Reclaim the Passion.

"Clarity of mind means clarity of passion, too: this is why a great and clear mind loves ardently and sees distinctly what it loves."

-Blaise Pascal

Finding Adventure in Change

While some nurses find a niche early in their careers and stick with it through their professional lives, Mary Schuett is among those whose passion for nursing derives from the adventure of constant change and new challenges. Her many-faceted career has given her a unique perspective. Sometimes the changes in her career stemmed from her need for stimulation and new challenges. Sometimes they were dictated by life's circumstances. But each change revealed nursing to be a profession that taps all sorts of talents in countless settings.

O ne of the things I value so much about nursing is the career flexibility it offers. No matter what I was doing in my personal life, I was able to find challenging nursing positions that fit my lifestyle.

When my husband and I moved to Ohio, we had planned that I would stay home with our two young children. My husband had just started a new business, and it didn't take an accounting degree to realize there would barely be enough money to pay the bills. After nine years in administration — and not having so much as taken a patient's blood pressure in years — I was more than a little insecure about plunging back into bedside nursing. But within twenty-four hours of my decision to return to work, I had three job offers and was able to start the very next morning.

I hadn't always intended to be a nurse. In fact, I started college with my sights set on physics or dental hygiene. But after taking a CNA course to secure a summer job, I was hooked. I have always loved nursing, but the best thing about it is never being tied to any one particular specialty. There are so many avenues that we can take, each offering challenges and rewards to satisfy any intellectual pursuit and fit nearly any lifestyle.

I started my nursing career at the University of Chicago on a med/surg unit and moved to neonatal intensive care (NICU) after one year. After several years in NICU, I worked in ICU at a community hospital in Fon Du Lac, WI, then started my journey into Long Term Care (LTC), where I have spent more than fifteen years. In addition to traditional bedside nursing, I have taught LPN students and CNAs, done consulting, worked in administration as a staff development coordinator and served as a director of nursing. No matter where I worked or what position I held, I always felt empowered to effect change and have an impact on the quality of life for my patients. That, in and of itself, is extremely gratifying.

When I think about the advantages of nursing, flexibility and diversity are always at the top of my list. My husband and I have three children and provided a foster home for a total of twenty-three children over eight years. I was able to balance my nursing goals with my family life by working night shifts in intensive care and rehab during the years we offered foster care. The balance allowed me to keep my nursing skills sharp and still be home for my family. Not many professions can offer that.

Having worked for two home medical equipment companies, I now train CNA's in incontinence care. As a clinical nurse manager, I travel the Midwest instructing nursing assistants in LTC facilities. Beyond teaching the physical issues related to incontinence, I help CNAs preserve dignity and maintain infection control standards. It's a new challenge that draws upon many of the skills I have acquired over the years.

My deepest appreciation for nursing's flexibility stems from a major personal event. Five years ago, I was critically injured in an auto accident, didn't walk for a full year and needed intensive rehabilitation. The rehab specialists felt I should avoid any work that would be physically taxing. Their solution was to offer to set me up with a telemarketing position, selling siding and windows. Instead, I phoned some contacts and, within a week, got a job as a director of nursing, despite showing up for the interview with a walker and a huge cast on my leg. This proved to me that even if you can't work with your feet, you can work with your brains, your smile and your heart. I used a scooter to get around at work for the first year and, even now, there are days when I need a walker. But I never had to leave nursing because of my physical challenges. I was hired for my experience and my passion for improving people's lives.

After the accident, I knew my choices were to be a handicapped person or a person with a handicap. At fifty, I just could not let a disability run my life. That experience added to my ability to deal one on one with patients who face life-altering trauma.

But even before the accident, I always valued finding ways to make patients' lives better in different settings. In NICU, it was bringing a newborn to a point where it would be healthy enough to go home, or working with frightened teenage moms so they could become comfortable bonding with a scary, fragile newborn.

In rehab, it was helping 70-year-old Mel accept his altered body image after having both legs amputated. One night I literally had to pick Mel up off the floor when he got up to go to the bathroom, forgetting that both his legs had been amputated three weeks earlier. He was trying to be what he deemed the "perfect patient", following orders, not making demands and accepting whatever information we presented without question. He didn't understand his rights as a patient. But I saw through his mask of stoicism.

Night shift is a great time to do patient teaching and to draw people out in conversation. I sat talking with Mel and waited for him to open up. Once he trusted me, he was able to express his fears about his sexuality and his role as a husband in the physical care of his family's home and yard. When he finally opened up, it was a deeply emotional experience. We both cried for his loss, yet we were able to move quickly into planning the next steps in his rehab and exploring prosthetics.

That night was a turning point for Mel and his wife. They have stayed in touch with me through Christmas cards and letters for more than a decade.

I have received immense satisfaction from every one of my nursing roles, no matter what my title, and have always felt passion for my work. Someone might look at my résumé and think I'm a job hopper. But that couldn't be further from the truth. When I have changed jobs it's been because I've been recruited and challenged with new opportunities to learn and grow. I love to try new things, and nursing lets me do that.

There's really no excuse for any nurse ever to be bored. Find your passion, take chances and work to improve people's lives, whether in a short-term medical unit or in a long-term residential setting. After twenty-nine years in nursing, I've been blessed with ample opportunities.

As told by:
Mary Schuett, RN, BSN, Clinical Nurse Manager

To think about and journal

Think about the many opportunities in nursing. Consider where you are today and make a list of all the different nursing roles you would like to play in the course of your career.

"A sense of humor can help you overlook the unattractive, tolerate the unpleasant, cope with the unex-pected, and smile through the unbearable."

–Moshe Waldoks

This Isn't Heaven, and I'm no Angel

Medicine can be serious business, particularly when we are dealing with life-threatening illness and injury. But there is also an abundance of opportunity to laugh with our patients and enjoy our time together. Finding light, humorous ways of dealing with the dour side of health-care is a gift. Linda Feeney Schroeder shared this example of how she used humor to help re-orient a patient in a kind, respectful, yet light manner.

One day I was caring for a middle-aged woman with a metabolic imbalance that caused her some intermittent confusion. When I entered her room wearing my white uniform she took one look at me and said, "I must be dead. There's an angel in my room."

Try as I might, there was no convincing her that I was no angel and she wasn't dead. After several attempts to reorient her, I thought it was hopeless. Just then, her lunch tray arrived, and it suddenly struck me how I could convince her that I was her nurse and she was not dead. I opened her tray cover and said, "If you were in Heaven, would you have spinach on your tray?" Strangely enough, it worked. She looked at that dark green glob and immediately knew she wasn't in Heaven, I wasn't an angel, and she was still alive.

As told by:
Linda Feeney-Schroeder, RN, MSN

"Don't cry because it's over, smile because it happened."

-Theodore Geisel (Dr. Seuss)

🕯️Never a Spectator

It takes unique qualities to be a nurse. Beyond the intellectual rigor, many nurses possess the capacity to do whatever it takes for their patients. Karen Early describes scenarios in which nurses stepped up to go the extra mile, not only for their patients but for other collateral victims of a crisis. The outcome is often enriching for both the nurse and the people we serve.

There are times when I feel so privileged to be able to participate in people's lives the way I can as a nurse. There have been many situations where I have been awestruck by the depth of and breadth of our professional experiences. Some are profound while others are just part of a day's work, but all of them matter to both our patients and the nurses who share the experience.

Several years ago, I was working as an ICU nurse. My 60-year-old patient, Jean, was dying, and we were doing what we could to keep her comfortable. Jean's four daughters were all present when she died, but they were not ready to leave. One of the daughters approached me and said she and her sisters needed time with their mother before the funeral home took her body. I think she may have been uncomfortable asking to stay in the ICU after her mother had already passed away, but it made perfect sense to me. I made sure that we had four chairs for the daughters to sit comfortably as they gathered around her bed, and I gave them as much privacy as I could so they would feel welcome to stay and talk.

Later, as the daughters were leaving, they told me how much it meant to them that I had allowed them that time together at their mother's bedside. It struck me then that what I had done had been a simple gesture from my perspective, but one that would give these young women a whole different memory about the day their mother died. We are often so involved in the intensity of our days at work that we forget what an honor it is to be included in some of life's most significant events. In that situation, I felt honored to play even a small role in such an important day.

Another day, just a few years ago, will also remain etched in my memory. There was a terrible motor vehicle accident involving about ten victims, which is enough to stretch any ER's resources. This being a small community hospital, we had to call in additional help immediately. Due to the weather, the helicopters couldn't airlift the critical patients to a trauma center, therefore, we needed to call in additional ground transport, too.

The accident occurred during a snow storm and involved several cars. Two out-of-state teens had been killed, and one of the critical victims was pregnant and ended up losing her baby. Another woman had suffered a severe head trauma.

In the midst of this controlled chaos, a local teacher who had been at the scene of the accident pulled up in a van with several children who had been in the accident . Though they were uninjured, there mother was critical. At that point, we were dealing with numerous issues. We employed our standard triage for dealing with the injuries, but we were also facing the emotional and physical needs of the uninjured children.

My colleagues all stepped up to the plate to help in any way they could. A few nurses actually took families home with them who had nowhere else to go. In the midst of all the arrangements, one of the nurses realized it was one child's birthday. She took up a collection for a gift and a small cake.

I don't think I've ever been prouder of my coworkers than I was that day. They simply rolled up their sleeves and did whatever was necessary to help the patients and their families. In a small community that is what we do, and that day was no exception. This caring atmosphere is one of the things that makes working in a community hospital so special.

As nurses, we have many privileged moments when we are allowed to share life-altering experiences with our patients and their families. It's really an honor and we need to remember that the seemingly simple choices we make in the course of a day's work can have a major impact on others. We can never take that for granted.

As told by:
Karen Early, RN

"How far you go in life depends on your being tender with the young, compassionate with the aged, sympathetic with the striving and tolerant of the weak and the strong – because someday you will have been all of these."

–George Washington Carver

⚱️Swallow Hard and Keep Going;

As an ER nurse for nearly two decades, Doug Egdorf has long ridden the emotional roller coaster on which we nurses so often find ourselves. With experience in both community hospitals and major trauma centers, his stories speak volumes about the kind of man he is and the gifts he brings to the profession. He reminds us of all the times that nurses have to swallow hard and just keep going during some of life's most difficult situations. We don't always have the answers, nor can we predict outcomes with 100% accuracy. But what we can do is embrace our work with the compassion and courage that it takes to do our very best for our patients.

No Time for Tears

E ven after more than two decades of working in emergency medicine, there are times when I question why I chose this line of work. There have been many days I've left work feeling that I'd barely had time to breathe, exhausted and thinking, "Well, the main thing is, at least no one died on my watch." Unfortunately, that is the nature of the work. The struggles we face as we help our patients through life-and-death situations are really roller coasters. Sometimes they defy the odds, and other times they leave us wondering what went wrong.

I was working in an ER/trauma center in New Orleans when I faced a horrifying situation. A young mother was about to run errands with her children, when she realized she had forgotten something. As she ran back into the house, one of the children climbed out of the car. Not realizing this upon her return, the mother put the car in reverse and backed over her young daughter.

I found myself not only dealing with the physical trauma to the child, but trying to console the distraught mother. Her anguish and feelings of blame were heart wrenching. Adding to my own distress, I had three young children of my own at home and couldn't begin to fathom how she must have felt.

The child died within an hour. I stayed with her and performed all the post mortem care needed. There was only so much I could do for the distraught mother, but I stayed with the family while their priest consoled them. My own grief was raw, yet I knew I couldn't break down, because I had to answer a call light in the next room.

Sometimes that's just how it is. Even though we might want to just sit down and cry, we have to keep it all together. There's another patient just around the corner with urgent needs too.

Taking the Bitter
With the Sweet

One night Jack, a 22-year-old victim of a motorcycle accident, was brought to our trauma center. He had severe injuries, and he arrested within moments of arriving. We did CPR for more than an hour, and I kept asking myself why; it seemed hopeless at best. Even when we miraculously got a pulse, I was sure Jack would be brain dead. He was moved to ICU on life support but died on the ventilator a few days later. I felt defeated, sensing that our work had all been for naught. It's often that way — heroics and struggle, only to end with death. After this instance, in particular, I found myself becoming extremely cynical. Why did we bother? Why did we fight the inevitable? Why did we put so much energy into something that was destined to fail in the long run?

But then we received a letter from the organ procurement program thanking for us for our efforts to revive Jack. The team said our quick intervention and persistence had preserved Jack's vital organs and now a man in Ohio had a new kidney, a woman in Illinois had sight-saving corneas, and a child in Florida had a heart, possibly enabling her to see her sixth birthday.

Here was the rainbow after the storm. Although Jack couldn't be saved, our efforts had made a difference in the lives of all of these other people. Part of my peace came from knowing that we had not only made a difference in the lives of each of the organ recipients, but more than likely they all had families and friends who would also breathe a sigh of relief that somewhere, someone had acted to grant their loved one a new lease on life.

God Only Knows

I had been working for several nights in a row. On the first night we had admitted Wendy, a teenager with renal colic, and sent her on to the med/surg unit with suspected kidney stones. Just two days later Wendy became severely septic and had to be transferred out. I found myself caring for Wendy for the second time in just three days, preparing her to be airlifted, and I think she was a bit relieved to see a familiar face among the group. I remember this little girl looking up at me and asking, "Doug, am I going to die?" Well to be honest, I didn't know how to answer. I didn't want to answer at all, but I said, "No, you're going to make it. Hang in there." I just wanted to give her a little hope. They always told us in school not to give our patients false hope, and I really don't. But sometimes that's all a patient has to hold onto. Wendy was so young, and it was just so hard to believe she wouldn't make it. She ended up spending six months in the hospital, and at times the specialists gave her no hope.

About a year later I was working at the desk in the ER when a girl walked up and asked if I remembered her. I knew she looked familiar but I didn't recognize Wendy at first. "You were the last person who spoke to me when I was being loaded onto the helicopter," she said. "You told me I was going to make it, and I believed you, and … here I am." I took away two important lessons from that case. The first is that sometimes the seemingly minor things turn major on us in a flash. And second, never lose hope. We're not God. We never know how things will turn out.

The Lost Farewell

Another incident in my career reminded me that we just don't know how much time a patient has left. While working on the med/surg unit, I was caring for a woman in her fifties with terminal breast cancer. While bathing her, I was trying to be as gentle as possible because I knew she was in pain. She was so fragile and yet so dignified and courageous in her battle. Her son was there, and wanting to give his mom some privacy during her bath, he asked if he could go to the cafeteria for lunch. I said yes, that his mom would be fine until he returned. But minutes later, I rolled her over to clean her and she died in my arms. He returned to find me holding his deceased mother. All he could say was, "I didn't get to say goodbye."

I felt terrible and told him how sorry I was. I had no inkling that she would be gone so fast. Four years later, the son showed up in the ER. I didn't recognize him at first, but he reminded me that I had cared for his mom while she was dying. Immediately, my remorse flooded back. I said, "Oh my God, I'm the one who told you that you could go to lunch." But he simply reached out to hug me and said, "Thanks for taking such good care of my mom." It was obvious that what he remembered about that day was far different from the heavy guilt I had laid upon myself. He recalled my compassion and tenderness toward his mother and all I could remember was that I was the one who had prevented him from being there when she died. We're often far too hard on ourselves.

Just as it's immediately rewarding to be part of life-saving efforts, it's horrible to face all of the many miseries we so often see as nurses. The abuse, the violence, the tragedies, the losses. We get tired. We burn out. But there are also many triumphs, many miracles to hang onto.

I get through it because I take a lot of pride in the work I do, and I always remember something that my dad once told me: "Doug, you don't have to like everyone, but you gotta love 'em." My dad didn't have an easy life, but he gave us some really invaluable gifts of endurance, compassion and strength. I take those gifts along with me every day.

As told by:
Doug Egdorf, RN, BSN

"There are many teachers who could ruin you. Before you know it, you could be a pale copy of this teacher or that teacher. You have to evolve on your own."

–Berenice Abbott

School Days

Every nurse can recall stories from his or her school days. Retired nurse, Ruth Saddlemire Faur, recalls an era of nursing education few of us ever experienced. The world she describes and the era in which she was educated and trained now seem as quaint as a dusty string of love beads in an old dresser drawer. But when she shares a sample of experiences that helped to shape the nurse and teacher she later became, we can easily recognize the same challenge that nursing educators face today in teaching students to honor the interpersonal, human aspects of healing as well as the technologies of medicine.

I attended a diploma nursing program in New York City from 1960 to 1963. In today's "anything goes" world, it's hard to believe we were once subjected to strict scrutiny on everything from our skirt length and curfew to when and where we could entertain boyfriends. We had formal teas every Friday afternoon, and as freshmen we had to learn and demonstrate the proper etiquette for serving tea. We were expected to attend chapel services five days a week and could only be excused once a month with a written excuse submitted to the Dean. We had to be properly groomed at all times but particularly for chapel. Even soiled shoelaces were grounds for reprimand. There was a mark on the wall indicating the regulated skirt length. Since the same mark was used for all of us, regardless of our height, this made for some interesting fashion statements.

There seemed to be rules for just about everything, as well as a hierarchy that was not to be questioned or disregarded. Freshmen were at the lowest rung of the hierarchy and were expected to give up their seats or their place on the elevator for upper classmen. We didn't find this strange or demeaning. As children of the Eisenhower era, we went along without questioning. It wasn't onerous; it was just a way of life.

The school cap was a really big deal back then. I'm embarrassed to confess this, but I actually chose my nursing school based on what the cap looked like. It was this tall, folded, crinoline job that was just the neatest thing. The capping ceremony was really a major event, and most of us couldn't wait to complete the first nine months so we could wear that cap. Unfortunately for me, I got capped and was immediately sent off to my OR rotation. I finally had the privilege of wearing my cap and here I was in scrubs. I felt ripped off, which might help explain why I did something totally out of character that day — something that gave me a little more to think about than my cap-less head.

I was in the back of the operating room counting sponges during a spinal fusion. This was a good place for me, since I was an extremely shy person back then. My back was turned to the surgical team when I heard the surgeon let out a profanity and a Kelly clamp went whizzing by me, just missing my head before hitting the wall. Incensed by the outburst, I picked the clamp up by the tip, marched over to the table, leaned over the sterile field and told the surgeon, "If you ever throw anything at me again, I will throw it right back at you." Glowering over his mask, he bellowed, "Young lady — outside!" I knew I was in deep trouble and was literally shaking. I think the rest of the surgical team sensed my impending doom as well.

Once out in the hall, the surgeon demanded my name, then said, "Well, Miss Saddlemire, you're right, and I apologize. I should not have lost my temper in there." From that day on, that surgeon requested that I assist him in the OR, and I ended up getting some great surgical experience.

But the human lesson I learned that day was just as important. I really shocked myself and everyone around me when I stood up to the surgeon, but it taught me something about self respect that served me well throughout my career: Nurses must learn to handle difficult personalities early in their careers or they will spend their lives walking on eggshells around intimidating physicians.

We had some really funny things happen in nursing school, though some of them could have been disastrous.

In the sixties, hospitals were still using glass IV bottles with screw-on tops, which enabled you to open them up with minimal effort. This was convenient if you needed to add a medication, but it also offered perilous opportunities to classmates who apparently had been absent the day common sense was parceled out. During a clinical, one such classmate was caring for a post-operative diabetic patient. His vital signs indicated that the patient was getting a little "shocky," so the doctor instructed the student to give the man orange juice. Realizing that the patient was NPO (nothing by mouth), the student began preparing to deliver the orange juice through the IV. Fortunately, an instructor intervened in the nick of time. I often wonder if that would have been the first case of pulp embolus in the history of medicine.

Blood was also delivered in glass bottles with screw-on caps. When one of the students was told to warm a pint of blood before administering it to a post-operative patient, she took a creative approach to the task. When I had entered the clean utility room for supplies, I spotted a stainless steel bowl on the electric hotplate. Bubbling away in the bowl next to an empty pint bottle was a hideous clot of blood. It was warm now, but I guarantee, it wasn't going anywhere near a patient. Not wanting to witness the wrath of the instructor or the supervisor, I turned on my heel and just kept a low profile for the rest of the day.

My experiences as a student served me well when I began teaching in the late seventies. I loved teaching the fundamentals of nursing to entry-level students, because the early courses provided a unique opportunity to imprint important values on impressionable minds. One lesson I always tried to relay to my students was to balance the art of nursing with the science. Students seem to be innately enamored with technology. The tubes, the machines and the challenges of understanding and then mastering all the equipment draw students like magnets to steel. Of course, that kind of knowledge is crucial. If technologies as rudimentary as IV bottles and blood storage can confound certain students, imagine what havoc they could wreak through ignorance of some of the more complex devices in our arsenal.

Still, technology is not the part of nursing that provides fulfillment over the long haul. I continually reminded students that all the devices and gadgets are pretty much the same from room to room, floor to floor and hospital to hospital. What is always unique is the person attached to the tube or the machine. I stressed that at the end of the day, their real rewards wouldn't be measured in how many tubes they inserted, but rather in recalling the people they cared for. It is the art of nursing, not the technology, that keeps us from burning out and reminds us that our work is vital.

Of course, there were times when I, too, got a bit burned out with my work, but I discovered early on that nurses must recognize the symptoms of burnout and actively seek ways to breathe new life into their own careers. There is a great deal riding on our success in doing so, because burnout doesn't just affect the individual nurse; it affects the patients, the families, our colleagues and, ultimately, the entire nursing profession. It keeps us from being the best that we can be.

I fear that the emphasis on technology is making nursing

so science-based that we're losing sight of the human elements of our profession. We cannot allow that to happen, because the nurse is often the only source of human interaction that patients get. The very soul of nursing is caring, respect and dignity. We need to communicate that more clearly to the public, because when we do, we speak volumes about our profession.

When I enter a room, it doesn't matter if I am in a uniform, scrubs or a business suit. I want people to know I'm a nurse by the way I treat them. Nurses represent dignity and care. It is because of those qualities that today, as I look back from retirement on a long and satisfying career, I realize that no matter what job I've held, I have always been proud to say, "I'm a nurse."

As told by:
Ruth Saddlemire Faur, RN, MS

To think about and journal

Think about some of the important moments during your education that helped to shape the nurse you would later become. Consider role models and instructors who made a difference. Were you taught to honor the interpersonal, human aspects of healing as well as the technologies of medicine? Several questions in the chapter, "Classes and Clinicals and Boards, Oh, My!" in Journaling to Reclaim the Passion will help you to recover some of the memories that were the foundation of your current self.

"No act of kindness, however small, is ever wasted."

–Aesop

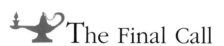

The Final Call

Where did we learn that professionalism means erecting boundaries between nurses and patients, no matter how much we may care about them as individuals? And how do we unlearn this? Nursing professor Suzanne Marnocha recalls an experience with a patient who taught her that such barriers are not only inappropriate but can actually degrade the most human aspects of nursing.

I was working twelve-hour shifts in intensive care, at a time we had twelve-hour partners. One of us worked twelve hours on day shift, and the other worked twelve hours on nights. One of my specialties in critical care was working with chronic obstructive pulmonary disease (COPD) long-term ventilator patients. I was the primary nurse for many such patients over the years and found that I grew very close to the patients and their families.

In Janet's case, I had become very close to both her and her husband. Early in her stay with us, Janet's husband brought in photos of the two of them when they were dating. It was obvious that he still saw her as the young, vibrant woman he had fallen in love with so many years before. Seeing those pictures was really helpful to us. So often nurses don't get to see the patient as a healthy, energetic person outside of the hospital bed and patient gown. Those pictures showed a side of Janet that would have never been obvious in her current condition. She was meticulously groomed and literally glowing with life in those photos.

One night after working my shift, my twelve-hour part-ner called me at home to let me know that Janet was dying and was asking for me. I thought it was such an honor that she wanted me with her. I knew her family well by that time, and I knew what really mattered to Janet.

I got to the hospital and got right to work with her. It certainly wasn't technical skills that Janet needed at that point. She needed someone to help her to say her good-byes with dignity. I was able to have her all cleaned up, hair washed and styled, by the time her family arrived. She had been bed ridden for so long that it was important to her that her family see her groomed and sitting upright for their final goodbyes. Janet's last ventilator episode had last-ed two weeks, so she hadn't been able to talk with her family during that entire time.

Being recumbent in bed is a powerless position, but Janet was such a vivacious woman, she didn't want to be remembered like that. She wanted to sit up in a chair, fully dressed, hair done, make-up on, with her feet planted firmly on the floor. Janet was meticulous about her finger-nails, so I made sure to paint her nails and help her with her lipstick. Once all that was done, she asked to be extu-bated so she could speak with her family and say goodbye from a position of full control.

Here she was, dying, and yet she was in control for the first time in a long time. Her daughter and husband were there with her when she passed away. It was a beautiful passing, and I felt so honored to be a part of their experi-ence. We maintained contact after Janet's death. In fact, Bill became a close personal friend over the following years. My husband and I even attended his wedding when he remarried.

One thing students struggle with is whether or not to get close to patients. So many nursing instructors tell students to avoid it, but I vehemently disagree. That closeness is part of the power of our profession. The closure we experience in saying goodbye is vital to us as human beings.

Somewhere, somehow, somebody thought it was a good idea to put up artificial boundaries under the guise of professionalism. We were trained to think that we don't need to get involved, to say goodbye or to grieve the loss of a patient. That is so wrong. We do need to go to funerals. And it is okay to grieve and to maintain relationships with families when appropriate. Commitment is a two-way street, and part of our professional responsibility is to put ourselves out there. Personally, I wouldn't have it any other way, because the commitment to our patients is what makes the nursing profession what it is.

As told by:
Suzanne Marnocha, RN MSN PhD CCRN,
Assistant Professor
University of Wisconsin, Oshkosh

"Love and compassion are necessities, not luxuries. Without them humanity cannot survive."

–Dalai Lama

An Emerging Image

How do we measure the value of a patient's dignity? Madonna Pralle discovered that in the end, respecting dignity disregards the pain, weakness and suffering we see before us in someone needing care. Instead, it honors the wholeness to which the patient aspires — not what we see with our eyes, but what we eventually see with our hearts.

I had been working in med/surg for several years when major construction forced our hospital to temporarily relocate and combine some services. For my med/surg staff, that meant accepting the AODA (alcohol and other drug addiction) patients onto our unit. As the nurse manager of the unit, I felt this was a logical move, so the resentment of some of my nursing team surprised me. Many of the nurses were impatient and often voiced disgust toward the AODA patients, particularly those undergoing detox.

Clearly, not every nurse has a desire to work with AODA patients, but even so, I was disturbed by how judgmental and opinionated some of my staff were in the beginning. I continually emphasized that our detox patients deserved our respect and that it was our job to preserve their dignity as they struggled through their recovery. I could have preached that sermon every day, and it would have fallen on deaf ears if it hadn't been for one patient who became the teacher the staff needed.

John was in his mid-thirties when he came to our unit for detox. A Native American from a nearby reservation, he appeared surprisingly strong and healthy considering his advanced alcoholism, but his hair was matted and disheveled, and he reeked of alcohol. Unaccustomed to dealing with alcoholism, one of the nurses openly voiced her disgust with his condition during report one morning. And though she always behaved appropriately in John's presence, I was disturbed by her response. I once again stressed the importance of preserving human dignity in all of our patient interactions.

I could sense that John was a proud man and embarrassed about his current state. He was always well mannered and seemed appreciative of the staff and me. Most importantly, he seemed committed to his recovery. He was a loner and spent much of his time walking the halls, wearing the same T-shirt every day while on our unit.

I never really paid attention to the image on the shirt until one day when he approached me in the hall. As he came nearer, I could make out the partially hidden image of a wolf among some trees. When I mentioned that I could make out the image when I focused a certain way, John smiled and explained that the wolf has important symbolism in his culture. He added that he had always related to the wolf's strength and self-sufficiency. As he talked of their similarities, I remember thinking that this was more aspiration than reality, because John certainly wasn't a symbol of strength and self-sufficiency at that point.

When it was time for John to be discharged, he stopped at the hospital gift shop and bought a small bag of chocolates for the nurses' station. As he presented the gift to me he apologized that he couldn't give us more. He explained that he didn't have much money, but he wanted to leave a gift as a token of his appreciation for the kindness and respect we had shown him when he was at his lowest. I found that to be a moving experience. The chocolates in themselves didn't mean nearly as much to us as the recognition and heart-felt appreciation expressed in that gesture. He truly was giving us all that he could.

The thing about working in detox was that we saw patients at their very worst, then usually didn't hear anything more about their progress or recovery once they were off of our unit. Seeing John reach even this level of recovery was such a gratifying experience for the nurses who had never worked with detox patients before.

About a year later I was working at the nurses' station when a handsome, well-groomed man approached the desk wearing a suit and tie, exuding professionalism and self-pride. When I asked this gentleman if I could help him, John re-introduced himself and once again thanked me for helping him through such a tough time the year before. Now, an executive with his tribe, he had fought his way back from the hell of alcoholism. To see him in such good health was a revelation, and I took the opportunity to call all the nurses to the desk to greet him. It was obvious that he needed to show us that he was much more than the disheveled wreck who had showed up on our unit only months earlier.

I think it was his pride that made him make that visit, but he'll never know what a rewarding experience it was for all of us. It's moments like these that confirm for me the value of our work. As John walked away that day, it dawned on me that he was, after all, very much like the wolf. He was strong. Yes, he had been lost and wandering for a while. But now, like the image on his shirt, he was coming back into focus.

As told by:
Madonna Pralle, RN

"Remember this — that there is a proper dignity and proportion to be observed in the performance of every act of life."

–Marcus Aurelius Anoninus

Maybe Today
I Made a Difference

There are so many times in nursing that we walk away from a patient encounter without even the smallest inkling that we have made an impact. Kim Udlis had one of those moments that has helped to rejuvenate her every day since.

That day was pretty much like every day for me in the cardiac care unit. I was prepping Dennis, a 48-year-old patient, for his third angioplasty when his cardiologist stopped in for his pre-op visit. He warned Dennis that if the procedure was unsuccessful, he would have to undergo open-heart surgery. Unfortunately, the angio failed and Dennis got the disappointing news. Knowing that he would probably be upset, I made it a point to spend some time with him. I sat on the edge of his bed and held his hand as our discussion moved from our shared love of hockey to his surgery. I told him how sorry I was that the angio hadn't worked and asked if there was anything that I could do for him.

Nothing about that encounter raised my eyebrow at first. In fact it seemed to be just another day interacting with patients the way I normally do. I would have never guessed the effect I had on Dennis until about two weeks later when this poem arrived in the mail. It happened to arrive on my birthday which made it even more special.

7/22/94
You came into my life uninvited
But welcomed.

At first just a friendly voice
in an unfriendly environment.
A tattoed, hockey-talking woman.
Nurse and patient.
But something happened.
Something clicked.
And in the blink of a butterfly's eye
we found something special.
Whatever that was, it was sealed in a dark room,
when in my sadness I reached out
and you took my hand and comforted me.
Once upon a time happens frequently in fairy tales
and infrequently in life.
And this is one of those times.
You touched my life,
Girl, dear.
And I'm the better for it.

"And I'm the better for it." That statement made such a profound impact on me and how I perceived my career as a nurse. I was so touched that he would take the time to write this poem and send it to me. It occurred to me that this particular day could have come and gone with the memory of our encounter fading like a flash. But this man made it a point to let me know how much my actions mattered. I called to thank him for the poem and he and his wife invited me to their home for dinner. They became a special connection for me over the years that followed. I've kept that poem in a frame in my office. It has moved with me along the path of my career since that day in 1994. When I'm fed up with patients, doctors and my crazy demanding schedule, I think of the poem and consider that maybe today I made a difference in someone's life and don't even know it.

Like every nurse, I have days when I ask myself why in the world I chose this profession. There have been times when I have considered returning to school for a career change, but then I think of Dennis' poem and it brings me back to why I chose nursing in the first place. His poem reminds me that I chose nursing over medicine or any other career because this type of interaction and memorable encounter is what is truly important to me.

Nurses can never take for granted the huge impact we have on the lives of our patients. When you add it all up – all of the nurses in all of the hospitals, clinics, assisted living, hospices and nursing homes – It is almost unfathomable the huge number of people we touch every day. We truly "touch" lives in aspects that no other profession can.

Nursing is so underrated, but some of that comes from us. We don't take the time to really reflect on the impact that we have. The media don't help either. Like the TV program **ER**. The nurses on that show who are really sharp end up going to medical school. What does that say about nursing? Although I complain, I watch it every week. Many in medicine and nursing do – for reasons similar to people gawking at a car wreck. In this case, we just have to see what they are going to muck up this week. The point is that we must not wait for others to empower us; we must empower ourselves.

I believe nursing is even misunderstood by some of our own educators. In nursing school, I took microbiology from a gruff professor with a thick accent. One day while working with me in the lab, he turned to me and said, "Noble (my maiden name), you smart kid; why you go into nursing? You going to do that til you have babies?" I thought how pathetic it was that this was how he viewed nursing. The smart ones only do it until they get married and have children. He was teaching nursing students, and this was the message he was sending.

Over ten years later, I have weathered the down times and stuck with nursing without regret. I went on to graduate school to obtain my masters degree in nursing and am currently working as an associate lecturer at a nursing school in addition to working as a family nurse practitioner. I really love my advanced practice. I volunteer at a community clinic for non-insured individuals in the Fox Cities (Wisconsin). It is incredibly gratifying because people are so grateful for the encounter, and you really get to reach the patients. Each day when I finish my work, I feel fulfilled, valued and truly appreciated.

Thank you, Dennis; you touched my life as well, and I am the better for it. And as for the gruff microbiology professor — I've had two children, and I am still proud to be a nurse, with many more years to come!

As told by:
Kimberly Udlis, RN, APNP

"Everyone should carefully observe which way his heart draws him, and then choose that way with all his strength."

–Hasidic Saying

♆Making the Dean's List

Today Anne Liners Brett is the Dean of Nursing at the Moraine Park Technical College in Wisconsin, but she wasn't always seated on that side of the desk. After a few run-ins with the Dean of Nursing during her undergraduate work, Anne nearly left the profession before she even got started. Fortunately, she breathed new life into her career and found that there really was another side to nursing.

I was an enthusiastic student, attending nursing school at a private Catholic women's college in Minnesota, when I had my first realization that I might not fit the proverbial nursing mold. In my second nursing clinical in a large teaching hospital affiliated with Mayo Clinic, I was caring for a woman who had just undergone an abdominal hysterectomy when in walked the chief resident with an entourage of medical students.

As every nurse knows, there is never any doubt about the pecking order for a nursing student. We were at the bottom looking up. So I wasn't particularly surprised when the chief resident ordered me to gather the supplies for a sterile dressing change. I dutifully returned with the proper supplies, which were handed off to one of the medical students, who proceeded to contaminate the field.

I was ordered to get a second set of dressing supplies, which were in turn handed off to a second medical student. Within seconds, the second medical student had contaminated the sterile field.

When the chief resident ordered me to get a third set, I was appalled but very calmly told him, "No, if your boys don't know how to do a sterile dressing, they should know where the supplies are kept." My first mistake was probably referring to them as "your boys," but my second, almost fatal mistake was saying this with our clinical instructor, Sister Greta, right outside the door.

Unfortunately for me, Sister Greta had impeccable hearing. She stood in the doorway, arms crossed, looking like she had just seen Satan himself. Without a word she pulled me aside and gave me two directives. One was, "You may leave now," and the second was, "Meet me in the Dean's office at 2 o'clock." My parents were called, and I was put on probation for insubordination.

I remember thinking that this wasn't what I had expected from nursing. I knew in my heart that nurses play a crucial role in patient care, and I was now discovering that they were sometimes treated like "gofers".

That was my first real disillusionment with nursing, and it had a real impact on me. But it wasn't the last time I was placed on probation for insubordination. The second time was when I refused to take part in a procedure I felt would be harmful to a patient.

Both of these incidents nearly halted my career before it got started and, by the time I graduated, I really wasn't sure that I wanted to be a nurse at all. With my once unwavering enthusiasm for nursing now shaky at best, I decided to earn a master's degree in educational psychology so I would have something to fall back on when I bailed out of nursing. I chose the mental health field because I felt it was one area where nurses seemed to be respected and valued. But then I started teaching, and everything changed.

It was only after I became a clinical instructor that I realized that nursing was exactly where I was meant to be. Seeing the practice through the students' eyes rekindled my excitement about the profession. Their enthusiasm and idealism helped me to rediscover nursing. By watching them grow and seeing them develop relationships with patients and with other nurses, I fell in love with nursing for the first time, and I developed a greater appreciation for the profession. Some of these students were kids right out of high school; others were in their sixties fulfilling a lifelong dream of becoming a nurse. I can honestly say I developed my commitment to nursing through my relationship with the students.

With my enthusiasm renewed, I went on to get a master's degree in nursing administration, then a Ph.D, I have always been a strong advocate for nursing, but my education and work in administration have strengthened my beliefs even more. I share my own student-nurse experiences with my students and encourage them to take pride in what they are and what they have to contribute. I continually stress that they are not "gofers"; they are intelligent, competent professionals with something to contribute, and they deserve respect.

I never realized the extent to which nurse advocacy had come to dominate my professional identity until one day when I was working with students in a clinical setting. I walked into the ICU behind a doctor. As he approached the nurse's station, one of the students started to get up so that the doctor could sit. The doctor put his hand on her shoulder and said, "Stay there. Anne is right behind me, and she'll kill you."

It is very encouraging to see how respected nursing has become over the course of my career. Today I am proud to say I am a nurse, and I am honored to be able to use my energy, skills and education to enhance the profession.

Sidebar

A few years ago I spoke at a Mayo Clinic research day for nurses. Much to my surprise, the former Dean (now a frail, elderly nun) from my alma mater was wheeled in to hear my presentation. Afterward, Sister approached the podium to speak with me. Much to my surprise, the same sinking feeling I had experienced in her office decades before returned to the pit of my stomach. Here I was with a Ph.D in nursing, a speaker at a professional conference, and I was cringing at the sight of this woman. I thought, "Get a grip, Anne." But the memories flooded back as she put it all into perspective for me. Pointing a wrinkled, shaky finger at me and with a look of true surprise, Sister said, "I remember you, Anne Liners. Look at you, we never expected you to make anything of yourself."

Her comment added weight to my opinion that I never did fit the mold back then. I'm glad to be in a position today where I encourage my students to break the mold as well. I hope that the new mold we are creating is one of value and respect — and has a much broader scope than the mold I helped break in the '70s.

As told by:
Anne Liners Brett, Ph.D., RN
Dean of Nursing, Moraine Park Technical College

To think about and journal

Anne Liners Brett found that she developed a much greater appreciation for nursing when she viewed the profession through her students' eyes. Have you ever taught another person a new skill or helped to orient a new employee? What did you learn when you became the teacher? Turn to "Teachers and Students" in <u>Journaling to Reclaim the Passion</u> *for further reflection.*

"Kindness is more important than wisdom, and the recognition of this is the beginning of wisdom."

-Theodore Isaac Rubin

A Second Wind

American demographics show that the average age of nursing professionals is forty-six. With demand for nurses increasing, the supply will dwindle rapidly unless the most experienced nurses delay retirement. As Lynn Dreson recounts here, nurses in their fifties and sixties may be inspired to work a bit longer if they can rekindle a deeper sense of purpose.

W orking in a peri-anesthesia care unit (PACU) since 1969 I have been able to witness vast changes in the practice. I have always enjoyed this type of nursing because every day is marked by a fresh set of patients and challenges.

We have the unique opportunity to deal with a wide scope of medical problems and surgeries that span the entire age continuum. But one of the down sides to PACU nursing in the past was that we didn't have interaction with families. We saw patients on their way into surgery and during the immediate recovery from anesthesia, but we didn't get to see them when they were well enough to be discharged. The truth is, years ago, families really weren't welcome in the PACU area. In fact, years ago, we nurses would resent it when doctors let parents into the PACU for children. Now I've grown to appreciate these encounters as opportunities to interact with families.

In the last few years, I was looking forward to retiring. In fact, I was, for the first time in my career, losing my enthusiasm and becoming tired of working. I had started to plan out my steps to retirement and was really beginning to look forward to it when I had a change of heart. I knew about the clinical ladder at my hospital as a way to increase my professional status and move up to the next pay grade. In the past when I investigated the required steps to become a Clinical Nurse II (CNII), I have to admit I was a little turned off. I thought, "Why should I have to prove myself with all of this paperwork and red tape? I know I am practicing at that level, so why should I have to do all that busy-work?" Then I took care of a patient who presented as a significant experience, and I decided to start the process. Once I started, my enthusiasm built and continues to do so. Now I have something more important to offer, and I challenge myself to give a little more.

I think my change of heart stems from two things specifically. One is the increased challenges I've embraced personally, and the other is that PACU has changed, allowing us more interaction with patients and families. In both regards, I am able to see more evidence that my work makes a difference.

As part of the criteria for becoming a CNII, I started serving as a preceptor. I have done that for an RN, two LPNs and a student nurse. I find that helping others to grow in their knowledge and confidence is very gratifying. Documenting evidence of my critical thinking via case studies has helped me to appreciate and articulate what I know. Sometimes nurses are so involved in day-to-day work activities that we don't give ourselves credit for the critical thinking we bring to the job. There's a lot of brain power in this profession.

Second, having more interaction with patients and families gives me a whole new perspective on my work. For example, I was taking care of an 18-year-old man who had hyperhydrosis (unusually sweaty palms). Embarrassed by his condition, Brandon had elected to have bilateral sympathectomy in order to eliminate the sweating. While filling out paperwork, Brandon confided that the reason he was having the surgery was that he felt he could never have a girlfriend because of his excessive sweating.

Despite his mother's reservations, Brandon proceeded with the surgery. Unfortunately, he bled excessively afterward. While his surgeon was completing other procedures, I needed to re-transfuse blood from the chest tube drain until he could go back to surgery to stop the bleeding.

Once Brandon was back from surgery, I called his mother who was in the family waiting area. I explained what was happening and forewarned her that he would be with me in PACU for some time. I could hear that she was crying, so as soon as I was able, I sought her out and found her pacing the hall. I took her back to PACU so she could see for herself that her son was okay. After that, I kept her posted with regular phone calls. Even when my shift ended, I stayed on just to make sure that she, Brandon and the family were comfortable and felt reassured. She was so grateful for my help that she introduced me to the whole family when I took Brandon back to his room after the surgery.

As nurses, we get a good feeling when we know we've made a difference. But it is especially gratifying when a family takes time to acknowledge us. It was almost a year later, during nurses' week, when I got a letter from Brandon's mom along with a photo of him at college. The letter said:

Dear Lynn,

You cannot begin to know how often we have said a "thank you" to you in our hearts, but in the crazy, busy schedules of our lives, we've not brought that to you first hand. In this time of honoring nurses, it seemed the perfect time to finally do so.

I hope you remember that day nine months ago and our son, Brandon. He had his bilateral sympathectomy (which I didn't want him to have in the first place!), and then started bleeding in recovery. I've no doubt I was in total denial of exactly how much danger he was in; and by the time he was out of the second surgery to repair the bleeding, I was exhausted and numb. You stayed with him every step of the way and — if I understood correctly — even hours past your scheduled shift. He remembers you as the one who talked him through it all. I remember you as the one who cared so deeply and was there for all of us! You are the best in the medical profession. I've worked in hospitals long enough to know how often that goes unrecognized.

We could never begin to tell you what you meant to us. I still get teary when I relive that day. Please use the enclosed gift certificate to get something just for you and know that it comes with heartfelt gratitude.

Examples like this serve to remind us that we're not just nurses working a shift and going through the motions of patient care. We're much more than that. Finding new challenges in my profession and really reaching out to others has given me my second wind in nursing. Before I retire, I would like to advance to a CNIII and take the national exam to become certified in PACU. With time and maturity, I've learned to let things roll off me more easily, and I'm gearing up for the next leg of the journey. In fact, I'm looking forward to it.

As told by:
Lynn Dreson, RN

To think about and journal

Have you ever been burned out with nursing? How do you find new challenges and maintain your enthusiasm? Turn to "Burn out" in Journaling to Reclaim the Passion for additional topics for reflection.

"*Whether one believes in a religion or not, and whether one believes in rebirth or not, there isn't anyone who doesn't appreciate kindness and compassion.*"

–Dalai Lama

Reaching Out from the Dark

At age thirty-one, with five children under the age of eight, Derry Bresee entered school to fulfill a lifelong dream of becoming a nurse. After graduation, she found her niche in home health and hospice care. Although Derry's clinical experience grew over time, she gained her greatest knowledge and gifts from a personal tragedy. In the process, she learned that there is no greater lesson for a nurse than shifting his or her perspective to the opposite side of the bed rail. It is only when we become patients ourselves that we truly understand the magnitude of the work we do. For Derry, it was her slow emersion from a traumatic coma that gave her the most valuable insight. Her near-death experience provides other nurses with lessons on the power of touch and the importance of being emotionally present for our patients, even when we think that they can't hear or understand us.

In 1997, I was in a car accident that put me into a coma for nearly three weeks. My last real conscious memory from the day of the accident was talking on my cell phone with my boss at the Hospice service where I worked. I had no recollection of the EMS extracting me and my son from the wreck or of any of the life-saving medical interventions that ensued. On the surface, to those around me, I was in a near-vegetative state, unresponsive except for basic reflexes.

Once my injuries were no longer considered life-threatening I was transferred out of the hospital and moved to a rehabilitation center but remained in a coma.

During those three weeks, in spite of my inability to communicate, I was able to read or sense the thoughts and feelings of the people around me. When the nurses touched me, I knew their thoughts and emotions by what was conveyed through their touch. I knew which ones were optimistic about my future and which ones considered me a vegetable. I knew which ones relayed love and healing thoughts and which ones were merely going through the motions.

I've always felt that communication skills are a vital asset for all nurses. But typically, when we think of communication skills, we focus on the written and spoken word rather than non-verbal communication, including touch.

I encourage nurses to use touch as one of the most crucial forms of communication. But even more vital than the act of laying hands on another human being, the real art of touch comes from being emotionally present and consciously imparting healing feelings to the other individual.

When you enter a patient's room, it is important that you put your mind and heart into a peaceful place. I recommend that you turn off any irritating and distracting noises like a TV or radio and prepare yourself emotionally to be with that patient. Leave all thoughts of problems, irritations and other patients outside the room. Consciously think healing, nurturing and empowering thoughts about your patients as you touch them. Even if they are not speaking or able to speak to you, they will feel your message. Above all, don't be afraid to touch a patient. When we don't touch our patients we are actually depriving them of a vital channel of communication. Human touch is the conduit for relaying our true thoughts and feelings.

When we lay our hands on our patients and consciously transfer our thoughts and feelings to them, we can reassure them about their physical recovery. It is also important that we reassure family members that it is good to touch the patient and to concentrate on positive and loving thoughts.

My coma was a near-death experience that allowed me to pick up on my nurses' thoughts and feelings. This personal tragedy has left me with an invaluable lesson for other nurses. If I could impart any bit of wisdom, it would be to convince them that as they care for others, they need to carefully and consciously channel their thoughts and feelings to their patients.

I was asked to speak at a March of Dimes, Nurse of the Year celebration to talk about my near-death experience. I wrote the following poem for the nurses to emphasize the power of touch:

Touch
I'm in a dark, dim place,
I hear sounds from afar off,
unintelligible sounds.
I can't understand the sounds!

I feel someone touching me,
moving me,
I know what they're feeling
when they touch me.

Do they know that what they're feeling
is communicated through their hands
to me, a near-dead comatose body?
Do they know that some part of my mind
is working, recording,
remembering?

I can feel that the person who's touching me now believes
I will live.
I KNOW I'm going to live,
LOOK!, I'm in here! I am alive!
I trust her much more
because I know she believes
I will live as well.

Do they know that they are communicating with me,
those who are touching me, caring for me?

I'm communicating the only way I can!
I'm in a dark, dim place,
hearing garbled noises from afar.
I don't remember who spoke to me,
I can't understand them!
I can't see them either!

But their touch,
that I DO remember.

It's difficult to describe my near-death experience. I remember watching my body from above. I could see myself lying in the bed with my husband seated beside me. I could read his thoughts and feel his intentions.

I have always believed in the power of prayer, but coming out of my coma I was conscious of the power of all the earthly prayers joined by a heavenly spirit. It was as though the earthly prayers intensified the heavenly prayers and I was surrounded by this incredible love and support that just lifted me up.

My physical disabilities won't allow me to work as a nurse anymore, but I still have important work to do. I regret not being able to work directly with patients but know I can contribute in other ways. I have written several poems about my near-death experience and have been interviewed a number of times about it. I have a personal mission now to help other nurses take more stock in the importance of being physically, emotionally and spiritually available to their patients. And touch is the most powerful conduit in that connection.

As told by:
Derry Bresee, RN
Hospice Nurse

To think about and journal

Sometimes touch is the most profound form of communication. Think of a time when someone has spoken volumes through a simple, well-timed touch. Reflect on any experiences that you have had as a patient. Turn to "Universal Language" in Journaling to Reclaim the Passion *for additional journaling ideas.*

"Goodness is the only investment that never fails."

–Henry David Thoreau

A Great Return on Investment

If we think of our careers as a part of an "emotional savings account," there are certainly many days when the withdrawals exceed the deposits. That is why we must bank the rewards of the profession — the life-changing epiphanies, the rich encounters, those rare, remarkable instances when healing seems more miracle than science. Each of these represents an opportunity to tuck away some emotional collateral that we can draw upon when life's rewards run dry. Lisbeth Cloute has been making spiritual deposits in her account for years. As a result, she has never doubted the wisdom of her investment in nursing.

I have been a nurse now for thirty years, and not a day goes by when I don't learn something new. It could be the latest in technology or some innovative drug therapy, but more often than not, it is a simple revelation about the human spirit.

During my career, I've worked all different shifts, but I always liked the evening shift the best. I enjoyed getting my patients ready for bed and giving them back rubs to help ease them into sleep.

These days, I have to wonder where that healing, nurturing philosophy and value have gone. About five years ago when my father had surgery, I discovered that part of nursing to be missing today. Though his overall care was great and the nurses were very skilled, I was struck by the fact that no one touched him for twenty-four hours after surgery; he literally had no physical contact. Nurses came in to check his pulse oximetry, NG tube, PCA pump and

IV, but no one laid a hand on him. The nurses even handed him disposable wash cloths so he could wash himself.

Today we have more technology than ever before, but it seems to be taking the place of human touch. When I think back on the simple practice of giving back-rubs, I realize it wasn't just the mechanics of the massage that mattered. That simple bedtime ritual communicated nurturing and caring to patients who were frightened, pained and vulnerable.

The dimensions of mind, body and spirit are all in need of healing, but we get side-tracked by the technology. Fortunately, I think we are starting to make a turn-around and beginning to value the whole person more, including the importance of human touch.

In my own case, I feel a spiritual as well as emotional and physical link with my patients. I can remember one particular child in the final stages of leukemia whose pain kept her from getting even brief sleep. I wanted so badly to comfort that little girl, but the medications were only marginally effective.

As I sat holding her on Christmas Eve, I rocked her and prayed that God would lift her pain so she could rest. I could feel her begin to relax, and for the first time in weeks she slept soundly. She died just two days later, but I believe that on that night, her peaceful rest was a gift from God.

I practice from a core belief that there is much more to healing than drugs, machines and lab tests. Every patient comes to us with a culture and history, and it's up to us to sift through all of their complexities in order to reach the healing place within them. An awareness of God's presence has helped me do that.

In recent years I have volunteered as a parish nurse, which had been a wonderful way to integrate my spiritual life with nursing. I think that family dynamics in our society have created a need for parish nursing because we no longer have extended families living together and caring for one another as they did in the past.

Our churches have become something of an extended family, and parish nursing enables nurses to practice within that community. A person may come in for what initially begins as a simple blood pressure check, but in the course of our visit I discover there is much more going on in their life.

I am able to serve as a resource person, educator and home visitation nurse for shut-ins. In this way, my nursing career has become a sort of personal ministry, because I am able to help others take care of themselves in the context of the church community.

For me, parish nursing is the essence of Shalom, which means peace or wholeness. Shalom incorporates spiritual wellbeing and harmony with God, and community. There are so many times when we cannot cure others, but we can heal them by sharing God's blessings and helping them to be the best that they can be.

My patients often thank me for the work I do, and I am completely humbled by their gratitude. It is I who should be grateful to them for what they give me with each and every encounter. I have gained so much more through my patients than I have ever given.

As told by:
Lisbeth Cloute, RN, BSN

To think about and journal

How do you incorporate your spiritual beliefs into your nursing practice? Have you ever faced conflicts between your personal beliefs and the job at hand?

Turn to the "Spiritually Speaking" section in <u>Journaling to Reclaim the Passion</u> and record your feelings about how nursing has contributed to your spiritual growth.

"Too often we underestimate the power of a touch, a smile, a kind word, a listening ear, an honest compliment or the smallest act of caring, all of which have the potential to turn a life around."

–Leo Buscaglia

The Power of Touch

Every hospital has something of an unspoken pecking order among their units and their nurses. Whether or not we admit it, that pecking order has a direct link to anthropology. Let me explain. When we use expressions like, "It's not brain surgery," what we are implying is that brain surgery is highly complex. Throughout history, the heart has been seen as the essence of life itself. When taken into a healthcare environment there is an assumption that the more complex the organ system and the care involved, the more skilled the professionals involved. Emergency departments, intensive care units, neurosurgery units and burn centers are among some of the most highly regarded units because many of the patients in these units are hanging in the balance between life and death. Nurses working in these units often relish the status of being among the elite lifesavers of the hospitals or "top dogs" as Tom Peterson describes them.

Tom Peterson will forever remember one patient encounter as a humbling experience and a reminder of the power of human touch. Most of us are exposed to human suffering in small doses as we progress through nursing school, but Tom received a bolus of life's most challenging moments before he ever took his first nursing course. The lessons he learned as a Vietnam corpsman served him well as he set his course in the nursing profession, evolving from a staff nurse to manager and now Vice President of Patient Care Services.

Tom shared one of his most life-changing moments, an incident that clearly shows the power of human touch as well as the need to stay in tune with a patient's emotional needs.

M arilyn was thirty-four years old and had been burned on over 80% of her body, nearly 50% of which were third-degree burns. Trapped in a house fire, she had heroically rescued all three of her children but had sustained painful and disfiguring burns that brought her into our burn unit.

Our team was the best in the business — or so we told ourselves. We were on top of the latest and most effective burn treatments. While other nurses just couldn't handle the stress of the burn unit for very long, a few of us were long-term diehards who could tough it out, no matter how difficult the situation. We were good, and we knew it. We had to be. Surrounded by some of the most intense pain, disfiguring wounds and the foul smell of charred flesh, the burn unit was no place for the faint-hearted.

When Marilyn arrived, we knew she'd be a challenge for us in many ways. We had a full team helping to manage her case, from social work to plastic surgery. We were on top of her pain management and even made sure that she spent time each day with her three children who were also patients on our unit.

Even a good day for Marilyn during the first three months of her five-month stay was never pain free. Since her burns were so extensive, there were only a few spots available for skin grafting on her buttocks and upper thigh. So the parts of her body that hadn't been burned were being sliced for grafts to the damaged areas.

Each day after working in a factory, Donny, Marilyn's husband of twelve years would stop in to visit Marilyn and the children. Donny was always pleasant and polite as he sat by his wife's side. More than once, I'd seen him glance self-consciously at the nurses when he'd lean over to give his wife a peck on the lips.

One night after Marilyn had been in the unit for three months, we were about to begin her bedtime routine of dressing changes and pain medications when she asked for something that shocked me to my core.

"Will you just hold me, Tom?" she asked with tears in her eyes. Totally shocked, I asked her what was going on. "No one has touched me, held me or even patted my hand for months. I'm hideous, gross and in pain. Even though no one should want to hold me, I need to be held." And with that she broke into heart-wrenching sobs.

Her words hit me in the gut like a shot-put. We had completely missed the boat on one of the main issues in her care — the healing of her spirit and psyche. Yes, we were managing her pain. We were successful in the skin grafts and infection prevention. We thought we were even helping to keep her family intact despite the fact that three of the four of them were severely injured and recovering.

Marilyn taught me that no matter how thorough we are with our clinical care of the body, we can never forget the powerful healing found in human touch. There are many diseases and injuries that can leave our patients with disfiguring changes. To help them cope with these life-altering changes, nurses can and should encourage family members and friends to touch, hold and remain close to their loved ones and to see past the surface disfigurement.

From that point on, our team made sure that Marilyn had privacy when her husband visited. We pulled the curtain to allow them to have private time together, and encouraged Donny to touch and hold Marilyn. We were reminded that she was not merely a burn patient but a human being with a husband, self esteem and the need for human touch.

In Vietnam, I had faced some of the greatest traumas

and human indignities known to man. There, it was my toughness that helped me survive. In my critical care experience I had been challenged by the technology and keeping up with the latest and greatest in therapies, and it was my intellectual capacity that helped me to stay on top. But what Marilyn taught me was that tenderness and compassion were even more important in her care than anything else. Her lessons will live with me forever.

As told by:
Tom Peterson, RN, Vice President Patient Services

To think about and journal

Have there been times that you completely missed a patient's most fundamental emotional needs? What did you learn from the patient? Turn to <u>Journaling to Reclaim the Passion</u> *and reflect on the questions listed in the "Listening" section.*

Don't Shoot!

Nursing jargon is a shorthand form of communication that we come to take for granted. It's one thing if we're tossing around terms in the nurses' lounge, but quite another when we use acronyms and arcane terminology in front of our patients. As Linda Feeney-Schroeder discovered, even the most commonly used nursing terms are inevitably going to be misunderstood when they fall on untrained ears. So, beware!

O ne day I was helping one of the nurses on the inpatient unit to get an IV started. The patient was a young man with tough veins. When I failed on my first attempt was to insert a twenty-gauge catheter, I said to the other nurse, "I'm going to have to get the twenty-two."

With a panicked look on his face, the young man said, "No, don't get the twenty-two. You don't have to shoot me. We'll get it in." Of course, being a small game hunter in rural Wisconsin, he thought I meant the .22 caliber rifle. We all got a good laugh over that, but it reminded us to watch our jargon around patients.

As told by:
Linda Feeney-Schroeder, RN

To think about and journal

How often do you use medical jargon in front of patients? What do you think this says to them?

"Kindness is more than deeds. It is an attitude, an expression, a look, a touch. It is anything that lifts another person."

–C. Neil Strait

⚱️A Universal Language

Compassion is contagious. The proof lies in the number of nursing careers inspired by a memorable childhood contact with a caring nurse. Dee Imai learned as an 11-year-old in Japan that the language of compassion is universal. Years later, as an adult in America, she became a link in the chain reaction of caring that has inspired nursing careers throughout the history of the profession.

I grew up in a small village in Okinawa, Japan, in the 1960s. We had no hospital; only a small clinic staffed by an old man who was not a doctor, although he'd had some medical training. Most of our health care services were delivered by American missionaries who visited our school and clinic to give immunizations and dental care. With such limited exposure to healthcare services, I never heard of a nurse until age eleven.

That was the year my new Dad took me to see a real doctor. I had suffered from chronic ear infections since birth and without access to medical care, I was not able to receive any real treatment until 1970. It was then that my mother married a US soldier, a wonderful man who took me to the military hospital. This first exposure to a hospital was my first encounter with nurses as well.

Since it was an American hospital, everyone spoke English. I had no one to translate for me other than my mother, who understood only a little of what was being said. But I was immediately taken by the way the nurses interacted with their patients. Their care and concern were obvious in their body language, facial expressions and tone of voice, all of which communicated kindness and compassion more than words ever could.

I was in the hospital for two weeks during that stay. I remember once in the middle of the night another young girl, around eight to ten years old, was admitted to my room. She was clearly distressed and was crying out in pain. I was awakened by her screaming, and I watched as the nurses touched her, held her and talked with her so gently, comforting both the little girl and her parents. When I couldn't get back to sleep, a male nurse sat at my bedside and, through signs and gestures, taught me to play a card game.

During that same hospital stay, a 2-year-old child was admitted to our unit in a spika cast. Understandably frustrated by her immobility, she needed more attention than the staff could give her. The nurses encouraged me to interact with the baby, and after watching how they communicated with her, I was able to mimic their care and compassion to nurture and comfort her baby.

I came to understand that being gentle and caring is a language that everyone can understand. The baby's family was so grateful for the time I spent with her that they visited me after my discharge and brought me a doll as a token of their gratitude.

That first hospital stay set my path in life. I knew I wanted to be just like the nurses who had cared for me and the other children on my unit. I decided right then that I would be a nurse, and I have never regretted my choice. Since 1981, I have worked with pediatric patients and their families, and I have had the privilege of recognizing that universal language in my own practice.

Over the past several years I have cared for a young man diagnosed with leukemia at the age of twelve. Mark is now in full remission, but returns to our unit for annual checkups. Always polite and cooperative, he thanked the nurses after each treatment and told us how much we had helped him. On his last visit, he told me that he is a sophomore in college and is majoring in nursing. It was his experience with us, he said, that had steered him to a nursing career. While he had always been impressed with our clinical skills, Mark said what had impressed him far more was that we had always treated him as a whole person, never as just a disease.

Later I realized that the lessons I learned all those years ago in Okinawa had come full circle. I had passed on the universal language of compassion. Now it is Mark's turn.

As told by:
Dee Imai, RN, BSN CPON
Hematology Oncology

To think about and journal

How do you reflect compassion without words? Turn to "Universal Language" in Journaling to Reclaim the Passion for questions to stimulate your thoughts.

"Oh God, help us not to despise or oppose what we do not understand."

—*William Penn*

Patient Advocacy

Being a true patient advocate takes guts and persistence. Sometimes the most exemplary nurses are the ones who stand up for patients' rights at all costs. Often the role of advocate is rewarding and fulfilling, but at other times it places wear and tear on us physically and emotionally — and not always with a positive outcome. Dr. Sharon Chappy was a classmate of mine at the University of Wisconsin-Madison. Today, she is a professor of nursing and shares this story with her own students as an example of the importance of being a patient advocate.

When I was a pretty new OR nurse I was assigned to transfer David, a man in his late forties, from the nursing unit to the OR for a PEG tube insertion. David was in the late stages of ALS and no longer able to swallow. I had heard from the floor nurses that he did not want this procedure performed and had expressed his wishes in writing. His daughter, however, had obtained a court order to exercise medical power of attorney and had insisted this procedure be done. Unfortunately for David, this was back in the days before living wills were commonly accepted. The court order was filed, and policy obliged us to follow through. I remember thinking that this was very odd since he seemed to be coherent.

After I wheeled David into the OR and was doing my last-minute checks, he gestured that he wanted to tell me something. I handed him a piece of paper and pencil and he scrawled out, "I hate what you are doing to me." He then went on to whisper very softly, "I just want to die. Please just let me die."

I was taken aback. For one thing, he seemed lucid, but for another, he was so adamant about his wishes. I immediately found his surgeon and described the dilemma. The surgeon basically shrugged it off and proceeded to scrub in, citing the court order. I felt awful and continued to press David's plea with the surgeon, saying I didn't feel this was right, yet I continued going through the motions, and finally did my part to insert the tube.

David was just lightly sedated for the insertion. I wheeled him into recovery, and I decided to sit with him myself until the sedation had worn off. As he became more alert, he overtly turned away from me, choosing to avoid eye contact. I tried to talk to him and he just looked away.

Thinking that maybe he was too weak to turn his head to look at me, I walked to the other side of the cart in hopes of making eye contact. He slowly turned his head the other direction to avoid my gaze.

As I sat there, I tried to think how I would feel if I were this man. I wondered if I would ever consider committing suicide if I had such a debilitating disease. Then I realized he was too weak to even carry out such an act. I realized this man knew what he wanted and no one had listened to him; first his daughter, then the judge and now the hospital team. Guilt overcame me as I realized I was a factor in prolonging his life against his wishes.

When I took him back to his room, I could no longer look at him. When I did, my eyes filled with tears. I felt that I had betrayed him.

He went home to the care of his daughter the next day. Three days later I saw his obituary in the paper. At the time, I wondered if he had found a way to end his own life, yet felt relieved that his suffering was over. To this day, I wish there had been a way to ask his forgiveness in not fighting harder for him.

David's lesson has stayed with me through all these years. From that day on, I have done everything in my power to ensure that my patients' wishes are followed. Although I am not always successful, I am much more assertive and will go to the source (often the family) to advocate for the patient.

I have realized that surgeons sometimes can be "partners in the crime" when avoiding uncomfortable confrontations with families. As nurses, we have a responsibility to listen to, and advocate for, our patients even when we might disagree. Sometimes the patient's only desire is that we do nothing at all, and that should be their own decision.

As a clinical instructor, I am able to share this story with my students. As distressing as it was for me on a personal level, I only hope that it gives my students the courage to stand up for their patients against adversity.

As told by:
Sharon Chappy, RN, PhD
University of Wisconsin-Oshkosh

To think about and journal

Consider any similar situations that you have encountered where you have felt frustrated by conflicting demands.

Turn to "Between a Rock and a Hard Place" in Journaling to Reclaim the Passion *for additional thought-provoking questions.*

"There are two ways of spreading light; to be the candle, or the mirror that reflects it."

-Edith Wharton

Holding up a Mirror

When someone holds up a mirror to us, we're forced to see ourselves as others do. With the help of a peer, Kathy Hageseth was able to reflect on her attitude and make a decision that was in her patient's best interest

About five years ago, I was caring for a young woman who was a victim of a crash involving a drunk driver. Both Denise and her husband, David, were ejected from their car and suffered multiple injuries. Both were admitted to our ICU in critical condition. David had multiple fractures but was conscious and had a good prognosis. Denise never regained consciousness and was removed from the ventilator two days after admission. She died with her parents at her side.

The young couple had only been married a short time before the accident, and our sense of tragedy deepened when we learned that David was the drunk driver who had caused the accident.

One can imagine how this fact had strained the relations between Denise's and David's relatives. While both families were devastated by the loss of Denise, there was the underlying sense of blame. And while it is always difficult to lose a loved one, it is even more tragic when the loss is caused by the actions of another person.

I was assigned to care for Denise while she was in the unit, which meant I was also caring for her family. As is common in these situations, I was bonding with the family and stayed with them through some of the worst moments, including the decision to take Denise off of the ventilator. Their decision was an agonizing one, and they showed courage and love for their daughter as they made the decision to let her go.

While I was bonding with Denise's family, I was becoming increasingly annoyed at David's family. How could they feel so sorry for him when he was the cause of all of this pain?

Our ICU follows a bereavement protocol that includes periodically contacting families after a loss. About three months after Denise's death, I called her family to follow up. I had a warm conversation with her mother who seemed very appreciative of our care, including the follow-up phone call. She did, however want to discuss something that had been weighing heavily on her mind.

She said that after the funeral, David had asked why she and her husband had decided to take Denise off the ventilator so soon. This question had caused her to doubt herself and the difficult decision to withdraw life-support. Not only was she suffering from the raw grief of losing a child, but now, she was surrounded by nagging self-doubt.

I talked with her at length about brain death in general and her daughter's situation in particular. I assured her that it was the head injury that ultimately caused Denise's death, not the removal of the ventilator. This information seemed to comfort her and dismiss her self-doubt.

When we hung up, I was furious. How dare David plant any additional seeds of guilt in this poor grieving mother! After all, it was he who had caused the accident!

I walked out into the ICU and described the conversation to one of my colleagues. She listened intently as I told her how angry I was at David's selfish, narrow-mindedness in questioning Denise's parents. When I finished, my counterpart gently reminded me that David had lost his wife. She further suggested that by allowing ourselves to place blame, we were leaving him out of our circle of bereavement support.

She was right. By passing judgment on this young husband, I was denying him the opportunity to benefit from the same level of support that I was giving to Denise's parents. Didn't he just lose his wife? Didn't he need and deserve the same support and compassion that I was showing Denise's parents?

My colleague's gentle admonition hit me like a ton of bricks. I had been denying David bereavement support, assigning blame and withholding anything that would provide him emotional comfort.

With a bit of martyrdom in the back of my mind I thought about calling David, but almost immediately I realized that I couldn't be the one to make that call. My own feelings would more than likely stand in the way of genuine, heart-felt support. And that wouldn't be fair to David's needs.

I asked the nurse who had cared for David during his stay in ICU if she would contact him. Although not a member of the bereavement team, I knew she could do a better job than me at that point.

That encounter taught me some invaluable lessons. The first is that all patients deserve the same standard of care, regardless of our personal feelings. The second is that as nurses, we have a responsibility to challenge and mentor one another when we see our peers slipping.

In this case, my colleague very respectfully held a mirror before me so that I could see the reflections of my own judgmental attitude. She could have allowed me to go on about the injustice of it all, but instead she challenged my view. This experience helped me to screen my thoughts and attitude and now I am far more likely to filter judgmental thoughts that could keep me from providing my patients with the best care.

As told by:
Kathy Hageseth, RN, BSN, CCRN

To think about and journal

Was there a time when you caught yourself being judgmental of a patient? Refer to the "Standing in Judgment" section in <u>Journaling to Reclaim the Passion</u> for further reflection.

"Develop a passion for learning. If you do, you will never cease to grow."

-Anthony J. D'Angelo

Touched by a Nurse

Nursing student, Karissa Ellis, is one of the "doers." When elected to the office of Breakthrough to Nursing Director in her state's Student Nurse's Association, Karissa spearheaded a program designed to attract youth to the nursing profession. Entitled "Touched by a Nurse," this program helps elementary, middle and high school students to gain a better understanding of the nursing profession. What started off as a simple idea, soon grabbed the attention of state and national health care organizations that were grappling with the issue of low enrollment and nursing shortages. Looking at the current shortage and the dismal projections for the future of nursing, Karissa decided that although she might not be able to stop the immediate hemorrhage, she and other nursing students could work to prevent a future bleed.

I didn't always see myself going into nursing, even though I grew up surrounded by nurses. From the age of four, my grandma encouraged me to become a nurse, telling me that I had all of the qualities that would make me successful. And who knew better than grandma? After all, she was a nurse — as were my mom, my great grandma and several aunts. I thought, "No way am I going to be a nurse. I want to be a lawyer, a teacher, anything else." Absolutely anything seemed more glamorous than nursing.

My love of high school chemistry led me into the pre-pharmacy program at the University of Wisconsin-Milwaukee. Although it was intellectually challenging, it didn't seem to meet my need for personal contact. I found that I wanted to interact with patients on a much more personal level than what pharmacy could offer. Still uncertain, I enrolled in an education program, thinking I should be a teacher. But Grandma never gave up. Every time I saw her she encouraged me more and more to go into nursing.

My mom, who was working in the lab at that time, encouraged me to get a job as a phlebotomist for a summer. I did, and I absolutely loved it – but the personal contact was still a bit limited. Of course, I could hone my skills at drawing blood and provide words of comfort, but I wanted to spend time with patients on the healing end of care and not just interact when I was poking them. I wanted to be there to help them. Grandma was right, and I was hooked. That fall I enrolled in a nursing program and have never regretted it.

As a junior, I was elected to the state Student Nurses Association. One of our goals was to help raise awareness about nursing as a possible future profession by visiting area elementary, middle and high schools.

As someone who grew up surrounded by nursing, I was sometimes amazed at how little most of the students knew about the profession. Many had no realistic exposure to nursing and only knew about the nursing actors they saw on TV!

During one visit to a middle school careers class I talked about the differences between doctors and nurses and about boys becoming nurses. One boy was very vocal about his beliefs in the traditional gender roles of male doctors and female nurses, and he had quite an eye opener when the teacher said that her husband was a nurse.

I always make it a point to talk about the diversity of the profession and how many opportunities are available regardless of the person's interests. I like to talk with the kids about the fact that I'll always have a job. Many of the children we speak to are from homes with parents who work in factories. They grow up not knowing about having a career with numerous options and I think this information will have an impact on many of them.

In teaching others about the nursing profession I have become even more committed to my purpose as a nurse. I hadn't realized just how passionate I was about nursing until a patient said, "If you're so smart, why don't you go all the way and become a doctor." That made me angry. I couldn't help but wonder, if this is the impression people have of nurses, what are school counselors and other key players saying to students?

When I describe the value of nursing to the kids, I talk about how many minutes per day a doctor spends with patients versus how many minutes the nurse spends with them. Many students have only been exposed to doctors, so I like to talk about the little-known professions of nurse practitioner and nurse anesthetist.

I have been amazed by the reaction to this program at the state level, which partnered with the state hospital association and the Nurses Coalition. We have been able to gain media exposure I never imagined. I never thought the program was cutting edge, but I was thrilled that it struck a chord with administration and has gained so much support. It feel good to hear from the schools we have visited and learned that, because of our presentation, there are kids who are interested in considering nursing as a potential career.

I cherish my experiences as a student. I cried when I saw a birth for the first time, absolutely overwhelmed by the experience. The day after witnessing the birth, I went into the mother's room and said, "I don't know how to thank you for letting me share in this." When patients let us into their lives in this way, they are giving us such a gift.

Another great experience involved a patient undergoing open heart surgery for a bypass and a valve. It was such a complicated surgery, and I had no other role than to be supportive. He was nervous, so I played some music to help calm him. I stayed with him throughout the entire surgery. It felt surreal and somewhat spiritual to be a part.

Beneath his tough façade, I knew how much he appreciated my presence. On his way into surgery, he thanked me and said, "It's so nice to know someone is here rooting for me." I was honored that I could be that comforting presence for him.

Through these and other experiences in nursing school, I have grown to appreciate many areas of nursing and will probably become a float nurse so I can work in all of them.

I know I am young and still a little starry-eyed about the profession, but I've already seen so many burned out nurses, and it's disturbing. Our patients deserve the best, and we have to be there for them.

For example, during a clinical, a family member asked why we were doing blood gases. I was shadowing a cranky old nurse who told them, "Because the doctor told us to."

I was surprised by her curt, dismissive response, so I patiently explained the value of blood gases as we weaned their father off the ventilator.

The nurse was really irritated with me and asked, "Why did you do that? Now they're going to ask a lot of questions." It was evident that she didn't want to be bothered. She was forgetting that we have a responsibility to the family.

I think one of the most important things I've learned so far in nursing is that we're not "just" nurses. We are teachers, chaplains and compassionate healers, not just a pill-pusher and bath-giver. I'm within a couple months of graduation now, and I can honestly say I am proud to be a nurse. I am grateful to the women in my life who saw in me the qualities that would make me a good nurse. I now see that I have a lot to offer.

As told by:
Karissa Ellis
Nursing student and Nurse Extern

"I think miracles exist in part as gifts and in part as clues that there is something beyond the flat world we see."

-Peggy Noonan

Miracles Sometimes Arrive in Tiny Packages

Nursing is often filled with surprises. Sometimes, regardless of what the textbook predicts, a patient defies the odds and expands what I call "the wide range of normal." For Eva Dye, a two-pound miracle broadened her scope more than she could have imagined, strengthening her conviction that her skills and compassion could truly make a difference.

Working in a special care nursery, I had become accustomed to seeing some of the most high-risk babies. In addition to caring for high-risk babies born to mothers in our hospital, our nursery was also a regional referral center for southern Wisconsin.

In December 2002, I was called in on my day off to help with a transport. We were responding to a call from a small community hospital regarding a woman whose labor was so advanced at twenty-eight weeks gestation that she could not be transported safely. So, on this cold December day, a neonatologist and I were rushed to the hospital about thirty miles away to assist with the high-risk newborn after delivery.

By the time we arrived, what had started out as a normal vaginal delivery had become a crash C-section. The baby was a chin presentation, causing her little neck to hyperextend, so pushing became nearly impossible. In addition, the cord had prolapsed, requiring emergency delivery.

In my own environment, I am vigilant and well prepared for such deliveries. But thrown into a new hospital with unfamiliar facilities, equipment and staff, I felt completely out of my element.

Any misgivings I may have had were quickly put to rest when baby Stephanie arrived. She weighed just over two pounds and was severely physically compromised. I remember thinking how tiny and frightening she looked. The trauma from pushing with her neck hyper-extended had broken blood vessels in her face, neck and shoulders, causing extensive bruising. This tiny new arrival looked like she had been through a battle.

The attending OB staff quickly stepped aside to let the neonatologist and me take over as the primary care providers. To stabilize the baby enough for transport, we intubated her and started an umbilical line. The hospital had no arterial blood gas machine, so we could only speculate about her true blood gases based on her vital signs.

As we raced her back to the special care nursery, the neonatologist and I were both fairly certain that Stephanie would not live. Her vital signs didn't inspire much hope, and her hematocrit was a mere fifteen. Her odds were slim to none and decreasing by the minute. I was mentally preparing to step into a bereavement support role with the parents, and I discussed this with my team at the hospital.

But when I arrived for my shift the next day, Stephanie had begun showing signs of improvement. Little by little, that tiny infant fought her way back. For the next two months, I took care of her each night that I worked, and watched her begin to strengthen and then to thrive. I felt that I was witnessing a true miracle.

When Stephanie was named the area poster child for the March of Dimes I was overcome with pride and gratitude that I had been able to play a role in giving this child a chance to beat the odds. She had been, and still is, the most critically ill infant I have dealt with in a transport situation. For me, the most gratifying thing about Stephanie's survival is knowing that my actions and skills had truly made a difference. But it was Stephanie who had defied our dour predictions and proved me wrong; miracles do happen.

As told by:
Eva Dye, RN MSN
Special Care Nursery

To think about and journal

Have there been times when you were shocked by a patient who surpassed his or her medical prognosis? How did these experiences help to shape your views about healing?

"Learn to get in touch with the silence within yourself, and know that everything in life has purpose. There are no mistakes, no coincidences; all events are blessings given to us to learn from."

–Elizabeth Kubler-Ross

Thank You, Howard

What makes each of us human and thus deserving of human dignity? LaVonda Hoover discovered her answer in a severely brain damaged infant with no hope of survival. When others persisted in treating the little boy like a breathing corpse, LaVonda made it her mission to bring love and dignity to the child's final days.

Early in my nursing career, I was working the night shift at a children's hospital in the Midwest. Beautiful little Howard arrived on my med/surg unit after spending his first five months of life in the NICU. His little body looked picture perfect with his pudgy cheeks and smooth brown skin.

Watching Howard sleep, no one would ever know the extent of his brain damage. Having suffered severe meconium aspiration during delivery, Howard had only minimal brain-stem function remaining.

This little cherub had been born to 14- and 15-year-old parents who had already given up on him. In the time that Howard was on our unit, I never once saw his parents or anyone else visit the little boy. I guess they had already said their goodbyes when they agreed that he should be a DNR (Do Not Resuscitate) while still in the NICU.

From the first time I saw him, I was in love with this little sweetie. Maybe I bonded with Howard because he had the same name as my brother, or maybe it was his beautiful face and perfect little body.

From the first time I laid eyes on him and heard his story, I knew that my real nursing care would come down to just holding him. Since he had no one else, I vowed I would hold, cuddle and kiss him and let him know that he mattered in this world.

On each of my shifts, I made sure that I was responsible for Howard. I would schedule my whole night to spend as much time with him as possible. There were no nursing assistants on the night shift, so I did all of his care, including respiratory aerosol treatments and percussion every four hours. Though I didn't have to, I always held Howard during the aerosol treatments. I would plan a block of time to just hold him and rock him.

All of Howard's nutrition was provided through a central line, so he didn't even require holding for his feedings. That was all the more reason to make the time to hold him as a part of his care. These were our cuddle times, when I would rock him, sing to him, and kiss those pudgy cheeks.

I was forever talking to him. I can't remember how many times I told him, "Mommy and Daddy said it would be alright if you went to sleep and didn't wake up." I really wanted to be holding him when he died so I could somehow communicate to him that he mattered to someone.

I always talk to my patients whether or not anyone else thinks that they can hear. I feel that communicating is a way of valuing another human being. No matter what level of brain function a machine detects, somehow the person's spirit knows that they are valued.

After a couple weeks on our unit, Howard started having brief episodes of apnea. Every time the apnea monitor went off, I went into his room to check on him, but each time I touched him, he'd start breathing again. After a few of these episodes, the doctor ordered that we remove the apnea monitor. I remember his words clearly. He felt it was a "needless charge" since we already knew that Howard was dying and he was a DNR.

Despite the doctor's order, I fought to leave the apnea monitor on. I wanted someone to be aware when he stopped breathing if for no other reason than so that we could simply hold him during his passing, caressing his cheeks and saying goodbye. I wanted his passing witnessed because he mattered to me. I argued with the doctor that we did need to know, not to resuscitate him but to make sure he didn't die alone. Technically I lost that argument, but on my shift the monitor stayed on.

One night my manager had asked me to switch my night shift to a day shift to orient nursing assistants. I agreed and punched in a little bit earlier in the morning than the normal 7 o'clock. As always, I stopped in Howard's room first to see him. But when I found his bed empty and unmade, my heart sank. His bed was stripped, but the light in the room was still on. I asked the night nurse where Howard was. "Oh", she said, "I wanted to be the one to tell you. I went in to give him his breathing treatment about 5:30 this morning and found him gone."

I hated those words. The apnea monitor had been off, and he had been "found." It was disgraceful. Little Howard deserved the dignity of having someone there when he passed away, but instead he was alone. His passing was not witnessed, but discovered. He was not held during his passing, only carried to the morgue afterward. His forehead and cheeks were not kissed as he went, only washed after he was gone. His parents didn't even want to come in to see him when we informed them of his death.

Howard may not have been aware of his surroundings, but I think we still owed him some basic human dignity. No matter the age, every human being deserves to die with dignity and in the company of another. This is a birthright.

In my own way I made a promise to Howard that day. I could only say that I was so sorry that I wasn't there and that he had to die alone, but I would try never to allow that to happen to anyone else.

Just 'being there' as someone passes away is an act of respect — a final gift that we can give our patients. Yes, it can take a toll on us emotionally, because it isn't easy, and maybe not every nurse is willing to do this. That's okay; it doesn't make you bad. But please take the responsibility to recruit someone else who is willing to take this role.

Since my experience with Howard, I have made sure that none of my patients died alone as long as I could help it. About four years ago, a friend was terminally ill and in the hospital. It was important to her family that someone be present to sit with her at all times so she wouldn't have to be alone, and I was asked to take part in her vigil. During one visit, I had been reading to her and talking with her, even though no one was sure she could hear. I was singing a hymn to her when she coded.

Looking back, I really think my willingness to sit with her as she passed away went back to my experience with Howard. I've often thanked that little baby for the important lesson that he taught me so early in my career. Because of the promise I made to little Howard, I have become comfortable enough with death that I can play this role for patients and families.

Although much of our nursing career is spent helping our patients and their families to recover or improve the quality of their lives, I have discovered a valuable gift in just being present as someone passes away. It's a small way that I can pay tribute to Howard and say, "You mattered to me."

As told by:
LaVonda Hoover RN, CPN
Pediatric Nurse, Medical Surgical

To think about and journal

Have there been times when the only support you could give to another person was simply your presence? What did you learn through the experience of just being there? Turn to "The Power of Your Presence" in Journaling to Reclaim the Passion, for additional thought-joggers.

"Judgments prevent us from seeing the good that lies beyond appearances."

–Dr. Wayne W. Dyer

⚱ Just One of Us

When 16-year-old Sheila arrived on the OB unit, Lisa Harris coached her through a difficult first birth and helped her learn essential infant care techniques. When it was time to discharge Sheila and her infant son, Lisa was less than optimistic about the parenting prognosis. She frequently dreaded sending those precious newborns home with teen mothers, particularly when there were extra red flags indicating a high likelihood of abuse or neglect. In Sheila's case the extra red flags included drug and alcohol abuse, a somewhat pampered up-bringing and divorced parents. When combined with the marginal bonding behaviors Sheila exhibited in the OB unit, Lisa had every reason to doubt what the future would hold for this mother and child.

A s a persistent patient advocate and change agent for maternal child health issues, I was among a group of OB and public health nurses who created an intensive home visitation program for high-risk mothers and infants in our community. The program, called Bright Beginnings, provides monthly home visits for the first year following delivery to support at-risk families. In addition to basic support, this program provides new parents accesses to many hopeful services and agencies.

Sheila was one of the patients I visited after her discharge from the OB unit. I felt certain when she left the hospital that she and her child were going to have a rough time at home. As a young mother myself, I knew how exhausting it was to juggle an infant and a job. In Sheila's case, that full time job would be high school and social life. I had seen it hundreds of times before.

I remember feeling a bit relieved as I saw Sheila's parents assisting her with the child care. I knew that this young mom would need support, and yet there is a balance between accepting support and taking full responsibility. In Sheila's case, I was able to watch as a very healthy balance was formed.

At first, I got the impression that Sheila did not want me making the home visits. I did my best to offer advice and encouragement, but she was extremely aloof toward me, to the point of being rude. If I'd been asked to describe her attitude at that point, I would have said she couldn't have cared less if I ever visited.

One day, I had to reschedule a home visit. When I called to let Sheila know that I couldn't make it for a week or so, I was really shocked that she seemed sincerely disappointed. She said she always looked forward to my visits, something I would never have guessed from her behavior. Most of our visits had felt strained for me, and I always thought Sheila was just going through the motions to prove that she was a fit mother.

That phone call was something of a turning point in our relationship. It had been the first inkling that Sheila was feeling a bit vulnerable in her new role as a mother. Because I had been investing a lot of emotional energy into our visits, Sheila's words meant a lot to me.

One afternoon, when the baby was about six months old, I got a glimpse of the kind of mother Sheila was becoming. My home visit was scheduled for an afternoon when Sheila was running in a track meet. I remembered thinking, Oh boy, here it comes. Another teen mom hitting a dose of reality trying to juggle an infant along with normal high school activities. But what I observed was a lesson for me.

I walked in and saw Sheila smiling and talking to the baby with loving attention, duffle bag packed and at the door, instructions written for the sitter. She was juggling school, sports and a baby — and she was succeeding.

I watched as Sheila fed her son, interacting with love and attention, then put him down for a nap. She had structured her afternoon to take care of her child yet be back at school and on the bus for a track meet by 3 PM.

I was amazed. Here was a girl I had assumed would never be able to handle the demands of motherhood, let alone provide a stimulating and nurturing environment for a baby, proving me completely wrong. As I watched her, I thought, my God! She's just one of us; a working mother who loves her baby and is struggling to keep her life in balance.

About five years after working with Sheila, I ran into her in a restaurant. She had not only finished high school but, she proudly told me, was finishing the nursing program at a local technical college. I was absolutely flabbergasted when she added, "I did this because of you, Lisa. I want to be just like you."

Frequently we discount the impact we have on our patients. In my line of work, I just do what I love and hope that a little of that love will rub off on my patients, but what I learned from this experience was actually two-fold. First, I became aware that I had been nurturing a negative stereotype about teenage mothers. After witnessing so many frustrating heartbreaks, I had begun to think the worst of all teen parents. I had always wondered why some nurses became bitter and judgmental. Now I had to ask myself if I was becoming one of them.

Second, I came to realize that I had really made an impact in someone's life on two levels. I had helped guide a young mom to a point where she began realizing her own strengths, gaining confidence in her new role. And I had been a positive professional role-model who inspired her to become a nurse herself. That was such a pleasant surprise for me. I guess my consistent presence over those first, critical months had sent a message to Sheila that I believed in her. God knows a teenage mother needs to feel someone believes in her, particularly when she is unsure of herself.

We can't expect our patients to always acknowledge our work. but every now and then I'm pleasantly surprised to rediscover that I can make a difference in someone's life. I had no idea when I first set eyes on that troubled 16-year-old, that I would not only help her cope but inspire her to find her own place in nursing. Who knows? Maybe someday Sheila will be that quiet, steady source of support for some other young girl struggling through her first difficult months of motherhood.

As told by:
Lisa Harris, RN
Director of Women's Services

To think about and journal

Have there been times when a patient has surprised you with a 180° turn from your original prognosis? How have similar situations helped you learn to suspend judgment of others? Has anyone ever told you that you are their role model? If so, how did that make you feel? Turn to "Unexpected Honors" in <u>Journaling to Reclaim the Passion</u> to explore this subject further.

"Kindness is more important than wisdom, and the recognition of this is the beginning of wisdom."

-Theodore Isaac Rubin

🪔 Bending the Rules

Nursing education is fraught with rules; hard-fast rules of infection control and clinical protocols are abundant. Of course these must be followed, but other rules that we encounter simply need to be broken (or at least bent) at times in order to meet the patient's social, emotional and psychological needs. Sheila Kun found the need to act on her patients' behalf and, in the process, found greater depth in her role as a nurse.

U nlike many of my colleagues, I never had "the calling" to become a nurse. In fact, my enrollment in nursing school was by sheer coincidence.

My psychology classmate, Rose, had decided to become a nurse. Since we carpooled together, I tagged along with her to the nursing department. Rose insisted that I would make a good studying companion and persuaded me to enroll. I was oblivious of what I wanted to do with my psychology degree so I thought, "why not?"

Despite the long waiting list, the Dean of Nursing was convinced that I would be a strong candidate and accepted me on the spot. Two years later, there I was, a new graduate nurse looking for a job. I lived only five blocks from Children's Hospital Los Angeles, so it was a convenient choice. It was a job, simply a means to support the family at a workplace close to home.

During my first year at Children's, I worked for the Laminar Air Flow Unit (LAFU), a four-bed unit with negative air pressure for reverse isolation. The patients on that unit had advance-stage cancer and required high doses of chemotherapy and needed the reversed isolation for their protection against infections.

We faced multiple challenges in caring for these young patients. Not only were they facing life-threatening illnesses; they were enduring severe side effects from chemotherapy and intense pain from bone marrow procedures. To top it off, they were dealing with the inevitable separation anxiety that comes from reverse isolation. These kids were literally cut off from human touch.

Food was sterilely prepared in jars and they were confined to a small room that was literally and figuratively sterile. Even their toys had to be sterilized before entering the room. These were the sacrifices in combating a deadly disease. No training had prepared me to help address their isolation, separation and tremendous anxiety.

Once I got into the profession, I wanted to do things for the patients in order to turn their mundane days into extraordinary days. At the same time, I had to deal with my own risk of burnout. It can be difficult facing all of the emotional issues we deal with day after day. I learned to ward off the burnout by telling myself, "one patient at a time" and to have a true passion for what I do.

In his book *In Search of Excellence* Tom Peters encourages the reader to look at companies and explore what makes them excellent. He emphasized that to be excellent, a company needs to pay attention to details and to know their business well. This was a philosophy that I was able to bring to my nursing career. Learning from Tom Peters, I decided to focus on a small area and become really good at it. I did that with my nursing career by focusing on pediatrics. Knowing this business well is more than acquiring and maintaining the technical skills. It is also about learning to read people and take risks when necessary.

One example of risk-taking that still makes me laugh after twenty years is a time when I helped a 12-year-old girl cope with depression from reverse isolation.

Tammie missed her family and her pet poodle terribly. But this was a LAFU, where all staff were required to wear sterile gowns in the room. No pets were allowed in the hospital, let alone in the LAFU. Yet Tammie's depression was so severe that we knew we had to do something.

A couple of us collaborated and decided to sneak her poodle, Sandy, into the unit in a small, brown bag. On the way to the unit during this covert operation, we bumped into the medical director of LAFU. I was petrified that Sandy would bark or move inside the bag and give us away. Holding my breath, we finally reached the fourth floor with the bag intact.

I suspect that the doctor knew what we were up to, but ignored the fact we were breaking the rules. It was all worth it when Tammie saw her furry visitor. Although she couldn't hold the dog, she was able to reach out through a portal and stroke him with gloved hands. The grin on her face was priceless.

Another time that I had to bend the rules was when I cared for a teenage girl facing a terminal brain tumor. Sonja had less than two months to live and confided in me that she was not ready to die and we bent all of the rules to send her home on a ventilator. At the end of her life she was on 100% Oxygen, which is just *not* done; a patient is usually admitted to the hospital when they require 40% oxygen. We had to overcome several obstacles in order to let Sonja have her wish to be at home as long as possible.

Death is such a scary subject. No one has training in facing it, so we felt we had to do whatever we could in helping Sonja through her last days. We got her situated at home with home health nurses. Once the home care was in place, Sonja's family was able to achieve a bit of normalcy. Sonja's mom was able to return to work and Sonja was able to have her friends around home as much as possible.

Sonja chose to return to the hospital during her final two days. During this brief stay, I learned that we really helped her to achieve a better quality of life and the sense of being in control during her final days. Sonja's experience taught me that we need to be there for our patients and families when they need us the most. When we put ourselves out there and go the extra mile, we earn a special place in people's hearts. Those families will remember us forever.

Having a real passion for nursing prevents burnout. I've learned to focus on what I *can* do to help my patients through this time rather than focusing on what I *cannot* do. Sometimes it seems bending rules makes all the difference.

I've been with LA Children's Hospital for over twenty-seven years now and wouldn't choose anything else. I've come to appreciate the unique role we play when we work with children. It allows creativity, respect, caring, knowledge and teamwork to be excellent at this job. Twenty-seven years after taking this job for convenience sake, I can say that I'm proud to be a pediatric nurse at heart, working for a great place that makes a difference in kids' lives.

As told by:
Sheila Kun, BSN, MS
Nurse Care Manager

To think about and journal

Have you ever faced a dilemma between the rules and a patient's needs? Turn to "Breaking the Rules" in Journaling to Reclaim the Passion for questions to stimulate your thoughts.

"With the gift of listening comes the gift of healing"

-*Catherine de Hueck*

⟐ Listening With the Heart

If all we hear when a patient speaks is the words he or she is saying, we may be missing the real meaning. Especially in moments of pain, stress and confusion, patients may be reaching deep into their subconscious experience to communicate in allegory or metaphor. Nursing professor Suzanne Marnocha first discovered this subconscious communication as a teenager, when her mother lay dying. It was reinforced later, as a young nurse, when she deciphered a young man's plea where others heard only confused babble. Today she teaches her students to look for deeper meaning instead of just words — to listen to patients with the heart.

When I was a student nurse I was assigned to work with a young man dying from leukemia. I remember walking into the room and meeting his wife, Monica, and thinking, "My God! She is so young to be losing her husband!"

Monica couldn't have been more than a year or two older than me, and I was dumbstruck to think she would soon be a widow. When I approached Jim's bed, I could see he was diaphoretic, pale, confused and restless. His sheets were twisted and damp, and he was periodically crying out. Monica was beside herself and clearly felt helpless.

"He keeps talking about getting out of bed and packing bags," Monica told me. "He's saying something about trying to catch the bus." I kept doing the prescribed nursing routine, measuring vital signs and making other assessments, but I soon realized that Monica needed more from me than Jim did at that point. Jim was confused. All Monica wanted was to soothe him, but he just couldn't be calmed.

I spent some time just talking with Monica, and between the two of us we realized that Jim was asking permission to pack his bags and finish his business in order to die. Our conversation became a deep bonding experience. Monica was feeling so powerless and scared. I couldn't begin to fathom what it was like for a couple so young to be facing such a painful parting, but I encouraged her to talk with Jim and gently let him know that his bags were packed and he was ready to leave. I knew instinctively that on some level he needed her permission to die. I asked Monica if she would like me to stay with her during his last hours, and I could tell she was relieved not have to face his death alone.

As Monica sat next to him with her own head sharing his pillow and whispering that it was okay to get on the bus, that he was all packed, Jim breathed his last breath. She later asked me how I knew this was what he needed. So I shared my own story with Monica and in doing so, I was able to soothe some of my own past grief.

When I was fifteen years old, my mom was dying, and in those days children weren't allowed in ICU. I was hardly a child, mind you. I think I had lived more in those fifteen years than many women do in thirty, but according to my birth certificate and hospital regulations, I was a kid. I remember finally being allowed into the ICU and seeing this cranky nurse in long white starched sleeves scurrying around my mother. Rolling her eyes, she said, "Your mom is out of her head. She's been talking about canning pickles all day today. Imagine that! Canning pickles!"

What I knew, even in my youth was that dreams project reality. Carl Jung writes about transpersonal images that have powerful meanings. This was a case in point. I could see that my mom was taking care of us even in her dreams as she prepared to die. She had spent her entire life caring for other people. Cooking, cleaning, sewing and canning were not just necessities for our survival but ways she showed that she loved us. Symbolically, I knew she was stocking the shelves for us, leaving behind the food and nurturing to care for us after she died.

I remember thinking how incredibly shallow this cranky old nurse was and how much she was missing by not really looking at her patients, not really seeing them or hearing what they were saying. She was clueless and insensitive to me and my mother. Somehow I just knew that my mom's making pickles was a metaphor for preparing to leave. Sitting with her during her final hours, I reassured my mother that the pickles were finished, the shelves were stocked, and I would be just fine. In our own way, we were giving each other permission to let go.

In teaching my own students today, I talk about powerful moments they have as nurses. Every time they have the privilege of being with someone in pain and in need, it is an intense spiritual experience. Even the smallest thing, such as sitting and listening, rubbing someone's back or even cleaning their room, is part of the spiritual experience. I use my own personal experiences to remind my students that their very presence is a bond, not to be taken for granted or discounted as insignificant.

As told by:
Suzanne Marnocha RN MSN Ph.D CCRN
Assistant Professor
University of Wisconsin-Oshkosh

"In order to succeed, your desire for success should be greater than your fear of failure."

-Bill Cosby

🕮 Olympic Moments

It's not always the major milestones that set our course in nursing. More often than not, it is the seemingly little things that cause us to stop, look over our shoulders and recognize just how far we've come.

Nursing school hadn't been an easy endeavor for me. Unlike many of my counterparts, I didn't enter the program right out of high school. Instead, I waited until the youngest of my three children entered school before pursuing my nursing education. But it wasn't the academics that made my nursing school experience difficult, it was the abusive manner of my clinical instructor during my final semester.

There was no mentoring or coaching, no warm words of encouragement, only demeaning and publicly critical encounters between this instructor and her students. I wasn't the only nursing student who became physically ill before each clinical in anticipation of her wrath. So the outcome of our final clinical was a group of new grads who lacked self esteem and any shred of confidence for critical, independent thinking.

Starting my first position as a new grad with no previous healthcare experience was overwhelming, to say the least. I think all the graduates who had survived the semester with the instructor-from-hell were starting our careers with self doubt and trepidation. Eight new grads started at the same time as me on a very busy forty-bed unit. Most of our patients required total care and were either in end-stage renal failure or end-stage cancer.

Looking back, I realize that my greatest struggle as a

new grad was learning to be an independent, critical thinker. I hadn't started nursing school with much confidence to begin with, and by the time I was through, what little I had remaining, had been stripped away. So the challenges I faced on this busy, total care unit made me question whether or not I had made the right choice in nursing. Then I met someone whose lesson taught me volumes about my role as a nurse.

Millie came to our unit from a home for developmentally disabled adults. She was agitated and screaming out constantly, obviously in pain but unable to communicate her needs. Millie had been in the hospital for days and, according to the nurse's notes and report, had been refusing to eat. She was becoming malnourished and dehydrated when I was assigned to her. The doctor caring for her was sure that we would have to place a feeding tube to prevent further deterioration.

When I first saw Millie, the dietary assistant was just leaving the room after plunking down her breakfast tray. Millie couldn't handle the utensils independently nor would she allow me to feed her. Each time I attempted to spoon-feed her, she knocked the food away screeching in agitation. Considering her restless state, I just couldn't imagine her doing well with a feeding tube, but I knew she had to start eating or we wouldn't have any other alternative but to insert the tube.

I don't know what made me think of this, but I took her tray away, spread a pad over her chest and literally poured the food onto the pad on her chest. Voraciously, she devoured two entire breakfasts. The tray and utensils had been too much for her and she was over stimulated by someone else feeding her. Needless to say, she was quite a sight to behold when her physician walked in. Here was Millie, propped up in bed, face covered in eggs with chunks of toast clinging to her make-shift bib.

The doctor's first reaction was horror seeing his patient covered in food. Before he could ask what was going on, I told him that she had just eaten two entire breakfasts and that I didn't think she would be needing a feeding tube after all. He was thrilled that she had eaten, by whatever means it took. Giving me a thumbs up and saying, "Clever, very clever," he turned and left the room.

Now I realize that this wasn't a monumental feat in the scope of nursing and medical practices, but it was for me as a new nurse. At that precise moment, a light bulb went off for me as I realized that I was Millie's nurse — her advocate. Meeting her at her level and solving a problem for her had proved to me that I could make decisions on her behalf. I suddenly realized that as her nurse I could order a special cup or utensil if I felt it would be best for her. I could act independently even if I was trying something that hadn't been tried before. I could be creative in problem solving for the patient's sake. And by God, no matter what my clinic instructor thought of me as a student, I was here now, in this room, making a difference for this woman who couldn't speak for herself.

I've been a nurse now for sixteen years, and I still think of Millie often as the impetus for my becoming an independent thinker and problem solver in my nursing practice. Millie made me realize that each of us is an individual with unique and valuable approaches to patient care. If Millie were here right now, I'd thank her for starting me on the path of self-confidence and critical thinking.

As told by:
Laurie Purtell, RN
Lead Nurse ICU

To think about and journal

Think back on challenges you overcame through creative solutions. What did you learn about yourself as you solved problems through your own innovation? Turn to "Art vs. Science" in <u>*Journaling to Reclaim the Passion,*</u> *for thought-joggers.*

"The fact that I can plant a seed and it becomes a flower, share a bit of knowledge and it becomes another's, smile at someone and receive a smile in return, are to me continual spiritual exercise."

–Leo Buscaglia

Just Being There
With a Smile

The smile is a truly a universal language. From six weeks of age we begin to smile as a means of acknowledgment and communication. Child development specialists have trumpeted the importance of that six-week milestone in maternal-infant bonding. But no matter what our age, a smile is an icebreaker, a sign of welcome and a signal that we are open and accepting of one another. However, sometimes as I talk with nurses about the importance of smiling in the overall scheme of customer service, they are offended. One nurse told me that it was condescending to remind nurses to smile. "We are professionals with serious jobs to do," she said, "and smiling isn't essential in patient care." I couldn't disagree more. As Linda Feeney-Schroeder discovered, it can be the most powerful tool in our repertoire.

One evening I was called to do an EKG, as the nursing supervisor often filled in for closed departments after hours. I went to the patient's room and met a lovely little gray-haired lady with an Irish brogue. I knew this was a preoperative EKG, but I didn't know what type of surgery she was having. As I began the EKG, she told me that she was from Ireland and that she was having brain surgery the next day. She was very frightened and although her daughter was arriving the next morning, she didn't have any family or friends around at the moment. We talked awhile, and as I left she seemed to be at peace. Then she said something I will never forget. "I was very frightened," she admitted, "but I am going to go to sleep remembering your sweet smile, and it will get me through the night. I'll be okay."

Afterward, I wondered what would have happened if I'd been having a busy or stressful night and hadn't smiled as I did her EKG. It was a very simple thing that seemed to mean so much to her. It made me feel so good to have helped her. It made me realize what a privilege it was to take care of these patients at such important times in their lives.

This little lady had given me much more than I had given her. I never heard what happened to her after that night, but that gray-haired Irish woman left an indelible impression on me. Whenever I think of her, I remember to smile, no matter how rough my day or how busy my shift.

As told by:
Linda Feeney-Schroeder, RN MSN

"Kind words can be short and easy to speak, but their echoes are truly endless."

–Mother Theresa

A Very Special Delivery

There's a unique bond that forms between nurses and their patients particularly when we share life's most memorable moments — both good and bad. Nurses like Kathy Smart possess the rare gift of knowing how to comfort a family who suffers the unimaginable loss of a newborn, leaving both altered by the experience.

Obstetrics is a place where about 99% of the days are happy ones for our patients. But when Jane and Martin came to our unit, it wasn't with the typical joy and anticipation that one would expect of a couple experiencing their fourth pregnancy. For them, it was a sudden, unexpected blow to learn that their child had died and would be delivered stillborn.

Jane had been scheduled for a C-section, consistent with her previous deliveries. But this time there was no joy, no anticipation, only a sense of dread. In such cases, our nursing role shifts completely into helping the couple cope with their loss.

I have found that couples in this situation need information as well as support. I tried my best to help Jane and Martin understand as much as possible about what was about to happen and what they could do to help. By doing this in advance of the delivery, we helped to lessen the shock and bring them to acceptance as gently as possible.

I explained that the baby would not have the pink skin that they would normally expect in a newborn and that she would feel cool to the touch. I told them that we would wrap the baby in a warm blanket and encourage them to hold the infant, explaining that couples who do not see and touch their babies will often have nightmares about the experience.

I asked if they had a name chosen for the baby and they did. With that information, I made it a point to call the baby by her name, Heather. By taking the extra time with the couple, I was helping them to anticipate each step and help them in their grieving process, bringing closure to the dreams that they had for Heather as a member of their family.

Jane had general anesthesia for the C-section which meant that Martin was the first to face the realities of their stillborn child. Once the baby was delivered, I escorted Martin into the nursery so that he could have private time with Heather. After wrapping Heather in a warm blanket to lessen the shock of her cold, lifeless body, I handed the infant to Martin and suggested that he spend time alone with her.

I encouraged Martin to really look at the baby by pointing out some of Heather's beautiful features. I find that this is important in making the whole ordeal real for the family. In this case, Martin was able to recognize features that made her look like her siblings. The hairline, the lips, the long fingers were all traits shared by his other children. Martin assisted me in taking Heather's footprints for the records and for a memory box that we prepare for families experiencing such a loss.

We'd all love it if every delivery resulted in a family leaving the hospital with a healthy newborn, but that just doesn't happen. We need to be sensitive to our patient's and families' needs and help them deal with whatever situation is at hand.

In our line of work we often don't know if we are making a difference; especially when a family is dealing with sudden, intense grief and shock. We don't expect patients to call us up and thank us for the work that we do, so we're often left wondering if we made an impact.

In this case, I am sure that the time I spent with Martin and Jane had a lasting effect on them. Their physician, as well as a couple of their family members, made a point to let me know that what I did that day made a real difference. Jane and Martin have stayed in touch with me for years after their loss, and I think we form a special bond with our patients when we share life-altering moments such as theirs.

As told by:
Kathy Smart, RNC
Obstetrics

To think about and journal

Reflect back on a time when the only comfort you could provide was with your presence. Write about that experience and turn to "The Power of Your Presence" in <u>*Journaling to Reclaim the Passion*</u> *for further reflection.*

"Laughter gives us distance. It allows us to step back from an event, deal with it and then move on."

–Bob Newhart

Who's Smiling Now?

Most nurses would agree that we share an appreciation for humor that is distinctly unique to our profession. There are things that we find funny that others might find disgusting or off-color. The reality of our work exposes us to some of the saddest, messiest and most distasteful functions of the human experience. I'm convinced that if we couldn't laugh, we'd burn out. It's often the silly, harmless mishaps like the one shared by Laverne Schauer that bring color to our busy days.

Eighty-seven-year-old George was no stranger to our med/surg unit. A colorful man with a toothless smile and shriveled gums, George was admitted a few times a year for dehydration. He had no family, so the nurses always spent extra time with him. Because he had no teeth, we gave him pureed food, built up his strength and sent him home, because he insisted he could handle independent living.

One morning after George had been with us a few days, I learned in report that he had died quietly in his sleep. The night nurse informed me that she had prepared the body and notified the funeral home. We were told that someone would be arriving to pick up the body within the hour.

George was in a double room, so the night nurse had discretely pulled the curtain attempting to shield the roommate and his wife from viewing the corpse. When I entered the room, the roommate's wife told me that she was helping her husband get ready for breakfast, but she could not find his teeth. The two of us combed the room and bathroom and even sorted through the linen bag to no avail. Baffled, the wife resigned herself to helping her husband gum through his breakfast until we could find the missing dentures.

Since the funeral home attendant would be arriving shortly, I thought I should make sure everything was ready for George's transfer. Stepping behind the curtain, I was horrified to see George with a huge, toothy grin. The dentures in his mouth looked outrageous in his tiny, wrinkled face with his shriveled gums. As discretely as possible, I removed the dentures and stepped out of the room. I could barely hold back my laughter long enough to make it to the nurses lounge.

After some thorough scrubbing and a vague explanation, I was able to return the teeth to their rightful owner. I'm sure that the image of George with this set of huge teeth will stay with me forever!

As told by:
Laverne Schauer, RN, Director of Surgical Services

"One's life has value so long as one attributes value to the life of another by means of love, friendship, indignation and compassion."

-*Simone de Beauvoir*

There Are No Boundaries in Goodbye

It's no secret that there is more to being an exceptional nurse than possessing good clinical skills. Nursing inevitably demands a balance between what we know and how much we care. Learning how to strike that balance can be difficult, particularly for nurses who work with terminal patients. As Dee Imai discovered, sometimes the professional boundaries get a little blurred, and that's okay.

Working in pediatric oncology, it goes without saying that we face a lot of loss and many sorrowful days. The nurses with whom I work are, for the most part, optimistic because the success rate is improving all the time. Today, we can say that 77% of childhood cancer is cured and our patients will grow to become adults. For the many who do survive, we have the opportunity to monitor their progress and cheer them on when we see them for their annual check-ups. Despite all the improved treatments, however, we still have to deal with loss on a regular basis.

Helping families to cope with the death of a child takes a lot of energy and compassion. Because our patients are chronic, we see them for long periods of time over several years. Due to the time we spend with each child, their families grow to trust us a great deal. The bonds that we form are strong, so when there is a loss, the nurses hurt too.

One incident in particular will stay with me forever. We were caring for a 2-year-old who had been in remission but suffered an unexpected relapse. Since she had come in as an outpatient for a routine follow-up, her relapse took us all by surprise.

The oncologist explained that we could give the baby treatment, but her chances were extremely slim. After sharing the prognosis with the parents, I stayed with them to answer any questions, then stepped out to allow them time to think and talk by themselves.

When I returned, the mom said to me through tears, "This is harder than telling you to take my own life, but we will let go and make her as comfortable as we can and make her remaining life as full as it can be."

Her words and her raw grief hit me hard on two levels. I, too, am a mother, and I couldn't imagine the pain of letting go of one of my children. But I was also the nurse who had cared for this baby over several months and numerous visits. I had shared the hard times with them as well as the hopes and triumphs. We had gone through the process together — patient, family and nurse. Now it was time to let go.

This was a time when I truly felt that I needed to attend the funeral. There are many rewards that come in forming deep relationships with families, but there is also the pain that we experience in a loss. Some nurses can get really hung up about professional boundaries and feel reluctant to attend funerals or reach out to families outside the clinical setting. If a nurse asks to attend a funeral service, I accommodate that. I may be short-staffed for three hours, but it's important.

Families have sought me out to tell me how much they appreciate seeing the nurses at their loved one's funerals. Over the many months that we interact as nurse, patient and family, our relationship is sealed. Attending a funeral demonstrates that we cared for a child far beyond our professional responsibilities. It shows the parents that we really loved the child and, at the same time, helps us with our own need for closure. Just being there offers us one more chance to comfort the family, to hug one another and to simply say, "You meant so much."

As nurses, we have a great opportunity to learn from our patients during their final days. It would be a shame for us to pass by the chance to live and grow through our work.

Seventeen-year-old Tara had lymphoma and wasn't ready to let go. She asked that we help her stay alive long enough for her to put some closure on her life. She was able to hang on for nearly two weeks before she died, just long enough for her to finish some important tasks.

Attending Tara's funeral was an uplifting experience for all of us. Two days before she died, she wrote letters to her friends and family assuring them that she was not afraid. She left numerous voice mail messages on all of her friend's cell phones saying, "I love you, and God loves you." Those words, coming from the lips and the heart of a dying child were so powerful.

Tara's family played her recorded messages at her memorial service. Although her breath was labored and her voice weak, her messages were clear. In her recording she told family and friends, "I'm not feeling great right now, and I know I don't have long. But please know that I am not afraid, and I will see you again. Stay close to God. He knows what you need."

During her memorial service, several of Tara's young friends read letters that she had written, and they talked about how she had inspired them. She always wanted her friends to be positive.

Tara had a beautiful singing voice. During a healthier period, she had recorded a CD which her family played as they showed photos of her life.

Attending Tara's funeral was an incredibly uplifting experience for me and the other nurses from our unit who attended. It helped us to put closure on this beautiful young life and reminded us that we got to be a part of that life in a very special and meaningful way.

As told by:
Dee Imai, RN, BSN CPON
Hematology Oncology

To think about and journal

Professional boundaries aren't something that can be prescribed. Think about times when you have struggled with boundaries. Write about these struggles.
Refer to the "Boundaries" section in Journaling to Reclaim the Passion for more thought-joggers.

"A teacher affects eternity. He can never tell where his influence stops."

-Henry Brooks Adams

🕯Here's Looking at You

We talk a lot about patient privacy in nursing. Mary Schuett learned firsthand the importance of proper introductions and getting patient consent before inviting students into a patient's private space.

I had been teaching LPN students at a local technical college while pregnant with my second child. Knowing I would give birth early in the second semester, I took a maternity leave from teaching.

After twenty hours of non-progressive labor, the doctor said it was time to rupture my membranes and left the room to get the necessary equipment.

The doctor returned with his giant "crochet hook" to rupture my membranes. His instrument of torture wasn't nearly as terrifying as what followed him into the room. Six pink-clad young women with very familiar faces sidled in after him. My entire LPN class was at the foot of my bed looking up my crotch! All I could do was cover my head with my pillow.

I guess my role as a teacher went above and beyond the call of duty that day. And I gained a new appreciation for getting patient permission to have students observe any procedure.

As told by:
Mary Schuett, RN, BSN
Clinical Nurse Manager

"*There are many truths of which the full meaning cannot be realized until personal experience has brought it home.*"

–John Stuart Mill

A Personal Ministry

Nursing education offers us a broad range of theory, but life teaches us the most valuable lessons. Kathie Friedel shared an important lesson about how her real life experiences put her educational theories into perspective.

After graduation at age thirty-two, I worked briefly in labor and delivery, then moved into long-term care and home health, and eventually returned to school to become a nurse practitioner (NP).

My NP emphasis was on geriatrics, which seemed logical since my personal life was quickly becoming immersed in the care of aging relatives. Both of my parents and my husband's parents were aging and in need of regular medical attention. Of course, being the "family nurse," I naturally stepped in as their advocate and frequent caregiver.

In graduate school, I focused my studies and my master's degree project on caregivers' relationships with their geriatric patients. The premise of my research was how a caregiver's behaviors and words cause elderly persons, particularly those with dementia, to become inappropriately dependent.

Many studies validated my thesis, which I came to see as an unequivocal truth. I was so confident, in fact, that I wrote and delivered in-services for certified nursing assistants (CNAs) on the subject. I felt that many of the caregiver behaviors were condescending, and I said as much. I was the expert. I had done the research. My brief, intermittent observations of the CNAs validated for me that their behaviors made the residents more dependent on them. It was not unusual to hear a CNA say, "Let me do that for you," rather than encouraging the residents to act for themselves. Eventually, I would discover that academic theory alone can not reveal truth.

What I lacked was the CNAs' hands-on experience as caregivers. My role in long-term care had been to give medication, to do treatments and to participate on teams orchestrating care plans, with none of the intense one-on-one interactions with our residents that the caregivers had.

That inexperience prevented me from allowing for alternative viewpoints, the most important of which was that there were situations in which dependence was the healthiest relationship between an aging patient and a caregiver.

The CNAs knew I was wrong. When I conducted their in-service training and stated my concerns about condescending words and behaviors, I could see from some of their expressions that several disagreed. But, since my perspective was well supported by research, I didn't bother delving into their views. Now, years later, I realize that they knew something I didn't know, and it taught me that there is a world of difference between academic theory and real-world practice.

Right after graduating from nursing school at age thirty-two, I married Tom, and it triggered a spiritual awakening. Turning away from an irresponsible lifestyle that had already resulted in two failed marriages, I seriously embraced Christianity. Tom and I took vows committing not only to each other but to the care of our parents as well.

I could already see that Tom's dad, Lindy, had an organic brain syndrome, and I willingly began to help with care-giving responsibilities. I went to all of his appointments with both his primary care physician and specialists.

I sought out a neurologist who could diagnose and treat his rare form of dementia. We even encouraged Tom's parents to build a home across the road from us, so we could better help with their daily care. My mother-in-law, Pat, brought in additional help to care for Lindy, but despite all our best efforts, he had to be admitted to a residential facility.

A short time later, we began seeing changes in Pat. Once a very social woman, she dropped out of everything she had once loved and began missing social engagements and appointments. Nurses at Lindy's residential facility shared my suspicions that Pat, too, was showing signs of dementia. Shortly before Lindy died, Pat was diagnosed with Alzheimer's.

Over time, Pat needed round-the-clock supervision, so I left a secure position as a nurse practitioner to care for her and to keep her as independent as possible. Before long, she moved in with us. Her Alzheimer's advanced quickly, and after a few dangerous accidents in the kitchen — melting utensils or forgetting things in the oven — it became clear that this once-gifted cook could no longer be trusted in the kitchen.

This really hurt her, but clearly cooking was something she simply couldn't do safely. She needed to be completely dependent on us for her meal preparation and, for her own safety, we needed for her to be afraid of cooking. That one criterion would determine whether she could stay in our home or have to live in a nursing home.

Suddenly, what the CNAs had known all along was becoming clear to me. At times it may be appropriate to encourage a degree of dependence, not just for the patient's own safety but for the sanity of the caregiver as well.

Pat's living with us has been a major life change for

Tom and me. Now, in our fifteenth consecutive year of caring for aging parents, our days are long, and our sleep is often interrupted. But we are living our vows to one another.

When I quit my job as a nurse practitioner, I can't tell you how many times I heard, "You are wasting your skills and education," but what better way to use my skills than to give one-on-one care?

I don't believe I could do this without God in my life. To stay centered, I get up early for time to pray and meditate before I start my caregiver duties each day. My abilities as a nurse give me the skill to give the proper care, but my passion for my presonal ministry gives me the desire to serve in this way.

Frankly, I'm hurt by people who say I'm wasting my education and professional experience, but I also cringe when they say that I'm a saint. I don't look at my life as though God dumped these people and responsibilities into my lap saying, "Here you go, now deal with it." Rather, I believe I have simply accepted God's invitation to join in His work.

The experience has also been a blessing professionally. I'm certainly becoming more confident, and after having lived this experience, I have so much to offer other caregivers.

Just as importantly, I have come to realize that real knowledge and understanding comes from a balance between research, textbook learning and the hands-on experience of being the caregiver 24/7. I only wish I could go back to my former CNAs and solicit the input I once so arrogantly ignored in creating my theory. They could have been the real teachers. I missed my chance to learn from their experience and wisdom.

As told by:
Kathie Friedel, RN, MSN

To think about and journal

Think about experiences that have helped shape your attitudes and beliefs. Reflect on ways that you incorporate your spiritual beliefs into your work. Turn to "Spiritually Speaking" in *Journaling to Reclaim the Passion* for further reflection.

A Pearl of Wisdom
From Teacher to Student

Suzanne Manocha, an assistant professor of nursing at the University of Wisconsin-Oshkosh shared this pearl of wisdom worth passing along.

I am forever hearing nurses complain that we are misunderstood or under-valued as professionals. I firmly believe in the power of word-of-mouth promotion. If nurses speak positively and enthusiastically about the profession, we are bound to generate more interest in and respect for nursing. I tell my students, "Learn what your passion in nursing is, and tell at least one other person."

I think if we all follow Suzanne's advice, there might not be a nursing shortage.

To think about and journal

How often do you speak enthusiastically about your work? Make a list of all of the things you love about being a nurse. Make it a habit to spend more time talking about the positive aspects of nursing rather than the negative.

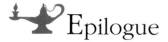

Epilogue

D espite the many hours spent gathering and writing these stories, the effort that produced this book never felt much like work to me. Part of the pleasure I took in the job derived from simply meeting such a diverse and inspiring group of colleagues.

It's no secret that nursing has long attracted remarkable people who approach their work with unusual fervor. Yet, amid the noise of our busy lives and careers, we too often grow calloused to the special nature of nursing and the special qualities of nurses. The stories of the men and women I interviewed for this book continually reminded me of that nature and those qualities.

Yet another reason this work brought me great joy is that setting these nurses' stories to paper gradually helped me to reclaim my own passion for nursing. The importance of that process cannot be overstated.

Because the work we do is the heart and soul of health care, we have an inspiring story to tell, both as individuals and as a profession. It's crucial that we share those stories so that all nurses can learn and grow vicariously through our collective experience.

Writing this collection has taught me that there is no one right way to rediscover the emotional kernel that fuels both the healing process and the professional life of a nurse. Tammie Heintzman found hers rooted in art. Kathie Friedel and Lisbeth Cloute found it in their religious beliefs. Derry Bresee, Dee Imai and Tom Peterson discovered it in the healing sensation of touch. It came to others in the form of relationships that sprang to life in an instant of human bonding and stretched traditional boundaries.

Yet, no matter where a nurse discovers a source of

passion, the very telling of these stories attests to the fact that reflecting on our work is a source of enormous energy.

This is why journaling is a vital exercise. Recording our memories, thoughts and feelings creates an outlet for our emotions as well as a personal chronology of some of our most important professional milestones and epiphanies. The culmination of our own histories will serve to rejuvenate us during times of disillusionment or fatigue. For that reason, I highly encourage you to continue mining the emotional foundations of nursing through personal journaling and group storytelling. Both are essential portals to self-discovery.

Finally, we should never hesitate to share our experiences with those outside the profession. The public image of nursing has matured greatly over the past two centuries, but we still struggle with shallow media stereotypes and popular misconceptions about the work we do and the value we bring to our communities.

These misconceptions won't be overcome by talking just to one another. To spread an understanding of our profession, we must evangelize. We must actively seek a more public voice. By sharing our stories with a wide audience, we bring honor to our profession, greater understanding to our patients and empowerment to nurses everywhere.

Kristin Baird
June 2004

Interviewed for this Book

Nurses interviewed for *Reclaiming the Passion* include:

Derry Bresee
Sharon Chappy
Sharon Chinn
Lisbeth Cloute
Lynn Dreson
Eva Dye
Karen Earley
Douglas Egdorf
Karissa Ellis
Linda Feeney-
  Schroeder
Karen Lee
  Fontaine

Kathie Friedel
Maureen Gosser
Kathy Hageseth
Lisa Harris
Tammie
  Heintzman
LaVonda Hoover
Dee Imai
Sheila Kun
Anne Liners Brett
Suzanne
  Marnocha
Tom Peterson

Madonna Pralle
Laurie Purtell
Ruth Saddlemire
  Faur
Laverne Schauer
Mary Schuett
Kathy Smart
Kimberly Udlis

Nurses interviewed for *Reclaiming the Passion* obtained their nursing education from the following schools:

Pacific Union College – Angwin, California
Cal State University – Los Angeles, California
Saint Elizabeth's Hospital – Lafayette, Indiana
Saint Luke's Hospitals – New York, New York
Lake Superior State University – Sault St. Marie, Michigan
College of Saint Scholastica – Deluth, Minnesota
University of Minnesota – Minneapolis/St.Paul, Minnesota
Saint Olaf College – Northfield, Minnesota
College of Saint Benedict – Saint Joseph, Minnesota
College of Saint Teresa – Winona, Minnesota
Lutheran Hospital School of Nursing – Saint Louis, Missouri
University of New Mexico – Albuqureque, New Mexico
Carolina's Medical Center – Charlotte, North Carolina
The Ohio State University School of Nursing – Columbus, Ohio
Vanderbilt University School of Nursing – Nashville, Tennessee
Weber State University – Ogden, Utah
University of Wisconsin – Eau Claire, Wisconsin
Bellin College of Nursing – Green Bay, Wisconsin
Northeast WI Technical College – Green Bay, Wisconsin
Saint Francis School of Nursing – LaCrosse, Wisconsin
Viterbo University – La Crosse, Wisconsin
Madison Area Technical College – Madison, Wisconsin
Saint Mary's School of Nursing – Madison, Wisconsin
University of Wisconsin – Madison, Wisconsin
Saint Joseph's School of Nursing – Marshfield, Wisconsin
University of Wisconsin – Milwaukee, Wisconsin

About the Companion Journal

Because of the emotional work nurses engage in every-day of their careers, I feel it is important to have an out-let of expression; a way to reflect on a day's work, the lessons learned and the lives we touch. For this reason, I have created a companion publication for this collection of stories, entitled *Journaling to Reclaim the Passion.*

In collecting stories for *Reclaiming the Passion*, I created questions or 'thought-joggers' specific to various sections of the book. This personal workbook/journal will help to recount experiences you may have had dealing with patients, family members, co-workers or professors and encourage you to look deeper into that experience to gain greater awareness about the situation and lessons learned.

At the end of selected stories in *Reclaiming the Passion*, you will see this icon: and a note asking you to refer to a specific section of *Journaling to Reclaim the Passion*. These selected stories have an important message to share and provide the opportunity for your reflection. It is in that specific section of *Journaling to Reclaim the Passion* that you will be given 'thought-joggers' or asked questions for further reflection.

When interviewing hospice nurse, Tammie Heintzman, (see "Music for the Soul" in *Reclaiming the Passion*) I had the privilege of sampling some of her piano music. Feeling so inspired by her compositions as I compiled Tammie's stories, I felt other nurses would benefit from her work as well. A CD of Tammie's original piano compositions is enclosed with every copy of *Journaling to Reclaim the Passion* for relaxation and inspiration.

I encourage you to listen to the music and reflect on the questions in the journal. Then, record your own memories, epiphanies and lessons that helped to shape you in your career and life.

Popular Presentations by Kristin Baird

Reclaiming the Passion — Celebrating the Essence of Nursing

This motivational presentation developed specifically for nurses will have you laughing, crying and re-affirming your commitment to the nursing profession. Baird uses storytelling about everyday people and the lessons they learned in trenches of the nursing profession. She reminds nurses to cherish their unique contributions and to reflect upon how their work shapes lives — including their own. This presentation is ideal for health care organizations that want to salute their nurses and celebrate the profession, whether it's through Nurses Day celebrations (May) or ongoing recruitment and retention initiatives.

Customer Service in Healthcare — Creating a Culture of Service Excellence

Based on personal experience, Baird shares steps to creating a service-centered culture in health care settings. Her witty, yet practical approach leaves her audiences spinning with take-home ideas for implementation. Baird takes her audiences through the common pitfalls of customer service programs and leaves them with a list of practical tips and feeling inspired to facilitate change. This presentation is appropriate for anyone working in health care. It is a popular program for helping employees at all levels of the organization to see their vital role in customer service.

Quality Through the Eyes of the Beholder — the Customer Service Link

Baird takes her audiences out of the traditional definitions of quality and helps them to see quality through the eyes of their customers. Using storytelling, skillfully combined with data, Baird demonstrates the link between service and a healthy bottom line. Baird encourages her audiences to embrace customer service at all levels of their organization. This presentation is appropriate for health care managers and senior leadership but can be tailored to other service industries as well. Components are used in a keynote or extended into a full day workshop. The full day workshop contains exercises to help participants hone the skills necessary in leading a service initiative within their own organization.

Kris Baird is an amazing speaker. She combines professional credibility, practical knowledge, humor, personal insight and effective speaking style into a very effective presentation. Ms Baird was the highlight of my Public Relations conference, receiving an "excellent" rating from every attendee.

– Kevin Stranberg
   Conference Planner, WHPRMS

Kris' interactive sessions were very well received and she sparked renewed enthusiasm for customer service.

– Tolly Arthur
   Director of Marketing
   Medical Associates Health Centers

I was so impressed with her presentation that I knew I wanted her to speak at our Iowa conference.

– Danice Larson, RN CPHQ
   President-Elect IAHQ

For more information about keynote presentations, speeches, workshops and consulting by Kristin Baird, please call Baird Consulting, Inc. at (920) 563-4684 or log onto
www.baird-consulting.com.

I have a passion for nursing!

Please contact me with more information on:

___ starting a storytelling group within my organization.
___ placing a bulk order of books/journals for my
organization's nurses. Discounts are available.
___ inviting Kristin Baird to speak at my organization.
___ placing me on your mailing list for information on
upcoming editions of *Reclaiming the Passion.*

* If you have checked any of the above, please provide the
following information for follow-up:
Name _____
Organization _____
Phone _____ E-mail _____
Address _____
City _____ State _____ Zip _____

Please submit this form by fax: (920) 563-3777 or by mail:
Golden Lamp Press, P.O. Box 622 Fort Atkinson, WI 53538

To place an order for *Reclaiming the Passion* or *Journaling to
Reclaim the Passion,* or to share your story, please long onto
www.reclaimingthepassion.com. For general information on
Kristin Baird and her work, please log onto:
www.baird-consulting.com.

Thanks for helping nurses to tell the stories of their great
work!

Order Form

Kristin Baird and Golden Lamp Press present...
Journaling to Reclaim the Passion – A Writing Guide for Nurses

- What first attracted you to nursing?
- What are some of the epiphanies you have experienced
  in your career?
- Who has been your greatest role model?
- What lessons have you learned and how have you grown
  through nursing?
- How do you overcome the "down times" in your career?
- Where do you find the greatest challenges?
- How can you tell when you have truly made a difference?

These are just a few of the memory joggers and writing cues that you will find in *Journaling to Reclaim the Passion.*

Every nurse needs time and an outlet for personal reflection. *Journaling to Reclaim the Passion* was created as a companion workbook/ journal to *Reclaiming the Passion – Stories that Celebrate the Essence of Nursing.* Beyond a collection of uplifting stories, the book and companion journal provide the reader with tools to reflect and articulate their feelings about the work that they do. The CD included with the journal offers a one-of-a-kind collection of piano music composed and performed by Registered Nurse, Tammie Heintzman. The inspirational music is designed to help promote a meditative, reflective mood for journaling.

Order Now!

(Please see next page for shipping and billing information)

Item Description	Quantity	Cost per unit	Subtotal
Reclaiming the Passion – Book (1 unit)		x $15.95	
Journaling to Reclaim the Passion – Journal/CD set (1 unit)		x $22.95	
Gift Set – Book, journal & music CD (1 unit)		x $35.00	
Subtotal			
Shipping & Handling		x $5.75/unit	
Total			

Method of Payment

☐ Check/ Money Order enclosed   ☐ Charge to:

❏ Master Card

❏ Visa

Card # _____

Expiration Date _____

_____
Signature of Card Holder

Order online with credit card at www.reclaimingthepassion.com.

Make checks payable to:
Golden Lamp Press, LLC

Mail orders to:
Golden Lamp Press
PO Box #622
Fort Atkinson, WI 53538

Ship to:

Name _____

Organization _____

Phone _____ E-mail _____

Address _____

City _____ State _____ Zip _____

Tell Us What You Think!

Dear friends,

This book came about through years of listening. Your feedback is valuable to future editions of *Reclaiming the Passion*. Please send us your comments and suggestions by copying and completing the brief questionnaire on the following pages. You may fax your completed form to: (920) 563-3777 or complete the survey online by logging onto:

www.reclaimingthepassion.com.

Thank you in advance for your support.

Kindest Regards,

Kristin Baird

Reader Feedback

To:
Kristin Baird, RN
Golden Lamp Press
P.O. Box 622
Fort Atkinson, WI 53538

Fax: (920) 563-3777
Email: info@reclaimingthepassion.com

From:

Name _____

Address _____

City _____ State _____ Zip _____

Phone _____ fax _____

e-mail _____

I became aware of *Reclaiming the Passion; Stories that Celebrate the Essence of Nursing* through:

❏ a friend's recommendation
❏ a web search
❏ a magazine/journal article
❏ other (please explain) _____

My favorite story was _____

I could relate to the story because _____

_____

One story that I did not care for was _____

I could not relate to it because _____

_____

I have a copy of *Journaling to Reclaim the Passion; a Writing Guide for Nurses*

❏ Yes   ❏ No
        If yes:
        • How useful is the journal (1 = not at all useful, 5 = very useful)

        1   2   3   4   5

On a scale of 1-5 please rate *Reclaiming the Passion; Stories that Celebrate the Essence of Nursing* on the following:

	Very Poor	Poor	Average	Good	Excellent
Quality of writing	1	2	3	4	5
Variety of stories	1	2	3	4	5
Balance of humor with serious stories	1	2	3	4	5
Writing cues for personal reflection	1	2	3	4	5
Use of inspirational quotes	1	2	3	4	5
Value received for the cost of the book	1	2	3	4	5
Value received for the cost of the journal	1	2	3	4	5

How likely are you to:

	Not at all likely	Somewhat likely	Not sure	Somewhat likely	Very likely
Recommend this book to a friend	1	2	3	4	5
Purchase future editions of *Reclaiming the passion*	1	2	3	4	5
Share one of your own stories	1	2	3	4	5

How could we have made the book better?

What would you like to see changed for future editions?